Eat Like A Buddha

Spiritual Recipes To Free Your Mind & Heal The World

By

SENSEI DEREK FLETCHER

EAT LIKE A BUDDHA

Spiritual Recipes To Free Your Mind & Heal The World

THIS PAGE INTENTIONALLY LEFT BLANK

CONTENTS

I.   Contemplation 1: The Self   1

II.   Contemplation 2: The Body   16

III. Contemplation 3: Nature   25

IV.   Contemplation 4: Universe   36

V.   Contemplation 5: Mind   48

VI.   Contemplation 6: Consciousness 70

VII. Contemplation 7: Integration   82

INTRODUCTION

This book had been percolating in my mind for two years before I actually sat down to "put pen to paper." As one opens up to ever deeper insights into the truth about all phenomena, most ideas and concepts become less useful as a practical matter. What increases is the direct experience of ultimate truth. One begins to see the subtlest of connections among all phenomena though these phenomena appear to be completely unrelated to each other. A wisdom unfolds that is far beyond mere understanding or academic information. Rather, it's a deep sense of direct experiential knowing that forever changes one's consciousness. Allow me to briefly share why I wrote this book and my unorthodox approach.

Once I was actually ready to fully commit to writing this book, I felt I needed to break the mold of my usual surroundings. This was not because those surroundings were insufficient to write this book. I simply sensed that this particular book needed to be written in an environment where I could be completely unobstructed in my flow of writing, thinking, contemplation and meditation. I also sensed that this book would be attempting to consolidate a massive spiritual matter into a concise and potent offering. This book was to be unlike any other book of recipes hitherto written. The essential ingredients here do not consist of herbs and spices. They consist of mind, Consciousness, phenomena, experience and wisdom.

I considered a number of places to go to write *Eat Like A Buddha*. After much consideration, I decided that I needed to leave the United States entirely, not just find a quiet spot in a remote area far from where I was living. Going to write in another state would also not serve this purpose. There were several personal milestones, such as completing my 50th revolution around the sun, that I knew could also impact the content of what I would eventually write. I wanted to remain relatively unknown, unseen and not be obligated to converse more often than necessary.

Weather, and being in nature, were also important in my decision on where to write. I wanted to open up completely to nature and its energetic power. I have had some profound experiences in and near bodies of water. So my choices were deeply influenced by my ability to regularly (as in daily if desired) go be with or in a body of water. I do not characterize myself as being an *animal lover*. But, I had dogs as pets growing up and loved them like family members. For this book, I felt for some reason which I'm unable to explain, that I also ought to be in closer proximity to animals. I suppose I felt it'd be more consistent with my desire to listen more than speak during this period.

Of course, food, language and cultural familiarity played some role in my thought process. However, they were quite minor compared to the degrees of solitude, silence, nature contact and energetic space I wanted. I nearly decided it would be Okinawa. Then at another point I considered India and then West Africa. Ultimately, based on a number of factors not particularly interesting or relevant to share, I decided on Riviera Maya in Mexico. It turned out to be a good decision.

Likewise, this move materialized the lifelong belief that I would at some point live outside of the United States. I have never known why or when that would happen. However, since my teenage years I have always deeply felt my life path would lead to spending more than just a few weeks or months in another land. So I eventually packed up my belongings and moved to Riviera Maya for a little over a year. I chose an area away from the hustle and bustle of downtown. Instead I opted for a suburb that was directly adjacent to a jungle.

I had the opportunity to see iguanas walking along the fence and sunbathing. Monkeys periodically jumped around in the trees. The birds provided a perpetual symphony of songs. Often I heard animal noises at night that I had never heard before in my entire life. Geckos and large red ants seemed to delight in inviting themselves inside. This was by no means an outback location. I did not desire that. I wanted food resources and other necessities to be within several miles of me. I chose not to have a car and walked 90% of the time wherever I went. I used public transportation, or my bicycle, to get to places further away. The walking aspect was a part of my overall desire to slow things way down and keep me extra disciplined about time. It also helped me get in rhythm with the movement of the sun.

But location was not the only factor I had to consider. I also knew that I needed time. A lot of time. I knew given both the subject matter of this book, and my approach to writing it, that I didn't want any artificial time constraints. I would need more time than it took to write my previously published books. In my mind I thought " I need a year to write this." A year sounds like an exorbitant amount of time to write a book. Perhaps it is. Especially to write a book that is "only" approximately 100 pages.

From my perspective, it was not just the book writing itself that required time, but the related spiritual practices, meditation and self experimentation I wanted to engage in while writing. We presently, live in a world of sound bites, 3 steps to success and 1 week to full enlightenment. I'm not from that school. I know my life practice has been one of discipline and willingness to stay around long enough to see what is fully present. I have learned that when it comes to spiritual knowing one must be willing to give to it whatever time is necessary. Fortunately, as a life long martial artist I don't struggle with efforts that may require weeks, months or years to experience the benefits.

So you may be wondering about these additional spiritual exercises and self experiments. I will share a few of them. One had to do with longs stints of silence, particularly not speaking unless absolutely necessary. Twenty to twenty five miles of walking each week. The goal with the walking was to readjust my physical rhythm to be more in alignment with the movement of the sun and my breath. Likewise, to observe how having a car creates appetites to "do things" that you'd otherwise go without if you had to walk. The time and energy wasted doing those things was shifted towards prayer, meditation and observing movements of my mind.

As I mentioned, meditation played a huge role in writing this book. I meditate daily as matter of personal practice and mind mastery. So meditating itself was not a change. However, my focus was often on something very particular. For example, I discuss in this book what food is. It is not what you would expect to hear. These meditations helped usher me through a 3 month dry fast. Essentially, my fast involved eating or drinking a minuscule amount of food, or nothing at all, each day. Please don't confuse this with intermittent fasting or time restricted eating. This is exceedingly more arduous and challenging than the strictest version of either of those processes.

I do not recommend that you try this without the guidance of an experienced practitioner as it could result in irreparable damage to your health or even death. I trusted that my years of fasting, meditation, martial arts training and mind mastery practice could carry me through and they did. I strictly adhered to the wisdom techniques I have used and learned over the course of my life. Eventually, I was able to go 22-23 hours without eating anything. I did drink 8 ounces of water once daily because I did not discontinue my martial arts training or other physical exercises. In fact, I increased them. Again, I do not advise you try this on your own.

There are many requirements to maintaining this practice. Meditation is a huge component of being able to do this without harming yourself. Part of the reason I needed solitude was I did not want to explain to friends, family members or other concerned parties, what I was doing. I did have the opportunity to see family members once in a while over videoconferencing. Also, I sporadically engaged with a few friends living locally. Each, in their own way, noticed my significant weight loss. Both family and friends inquired without prying simply by asking if "I was ok." Alternatively, they sometimes asked: "Are you losing weight?" I would just answer "yes" and change the subject.

I knew as part of this experiment weight loss (perhaps significant) would be a part of it. It was not a goal or intention. I knew what they were hinting at. When you start to see the physical body go through such substantial change it can be utterly terrifying. One must be a highly seasoned meditation practitioner, possess a deep understanding of the mind and know how to tap into energy sources available to the body that does not include food. You'll learn all about these other sources in one of the contemplations in this book. The lack of a strong meditation discipline, insufficient understanding of non-conventional food energy sources coupled with an extreme attachment to a false notion of a "self" puts spiritual practice of this kind far beyond most people's reach.

The fact is, I felt wonderful. Vibrant and clear in ways that words can't capture. I learned first hand how food as a phenomenon becomes a lifelong distraction for most people. Most people can't imagine a day that is not scheduled around eating conventional food…or not eating at all. I shall share more about this fasting experience, and related spiritual exercises, in the audio companion to this book. For now, let us turn finally to the approach I took to writing this book.

I took an unconventional approach to writing *Eat Like A Buddha*. It is a book of several extensive contemplations in which myriad other sub-contemplative pearls are also present. I have attempted to capture my literal contemplative journey along with its accompanying mind movements. What is presented here has been written from a certain level of consciousness that is the result of 3 ingredients. My life-long practice of self-discipline, the primed physical and psychological states I intentionally created while writing this book and the real-time contemplative insights they produced. I discarded anything from these pages that did not arise directly from the contemplative journey itself.

The goal is for you to get an inside look into the deep recesses of the consciousness of one being's intense contemplative journey. I believe I was successful at achieving this. There are undoubtedly some revelations shared here that may be quite challenging to understand. I kept them all. In order for you to get access to something of a completely different order of organic thought, I could not discard them. I could not omit anything because I thought the reader might not understand. I trusted that my contemplative process "as is" would be the most potent and authentic gift I could share.

Finally, a word on how to read this book. It is a book of contemplations. Read it slowly…very slowly. Though it is relatively short in number of pages, the weight is significant. You may benefit from reading a few lines or paragraphs at a time then stop to reflect before continuing. Take the opportunity to simply follow what is presented without adding your own mind's content. Just observe the reflections, questioning and unfolding of another being's free unobstructed exploration. After your first reading is completed, take up each contemplation individually on your own during the second reading. Experientially verify your truth about food and then methodically implement new eating practices that are harmonious with your new enlightened knowing.

CONTEMPLATION #1: The Self

*To believe you are a self, or that you have self, is to create
the greatest barrier to full Awareness.*

~Sensei

At first glance, in what you refer to as your "self" is where you think the most intimate form of communication takes place. However, we shall discover together, in this first contemplation that this is not true. To experience unobstructed universal communication one must first be liberated from acquired and inherited limitations and identities. One who is either unable or unwilling to do this will necessarily be extremely limited in what he or she can conceive, interpret, experience or understand. Let's first dive more deeply into what is meant by acquired versus inherited limitations and identities.

"Acquired" limitations and identities are **all** concepts, speech, thoughts and actions that an individual engages in to create and maintain a separateness called "self." These efforts are primarily designed to show one's difference from all other phenomena and especially other people. I am of the opinion that this sole activity is what the majority of humans spend their short existence doing. One is constantly in a state of measuring and comparing his or her own health, beauty, success, characteristics, abilities and accomplishments against others. If you feel you excel others in any situation you become prideful and believe you are happy. When you feel you are being outdone you become sad, angry, jealous or perhaps envious.

Whether you believe you excel others, or are bested by them, in both cases two false categories are created: self and other. In this business of "making self-known-and-separate" human beings fail to realize that they are simultaneously cutting themselves off from full Awareness. Herein lies the hidden poison of self-making. It is in every sense a fall from grace. It is to erect a perpetual prison fortified by the very concepts, thoughts, speech and actions intentionally used to create and maintain this self.

People engaged in the self-making process believe they are in a dialogue. That is, the more you believe in the false appearance you are creating (i.e a self) the more you believe that you are in conversation with this other you've created. We may now see the next level of deception in this process. The more a human being creates a false appearance of self-and-other the more "things" they believe there are to be desired, feared, owned, used or abused. The truth is that with each additional instance of otherizing the false appearance of self becomes more divided and alienated. One believes to the degree I am "this" (a self) I am necessarily not "that." (any other thing) So the ongoing conversation in the mind is strictly about self-and-other. It appears to be a dialogue. Still, a fully Aware being knows no division.

Note today the extreme lengths people go to show how different they are from others and how everyone else must acknowledge and respect that difference. They demand that you recognize they are a "such-and-such" or "so-and-so." Any other self that disagrees with this becomes an enemy-other. Any other self that agrees or supports this difference becomes an ally-other. In either case, separation and difference are at the root of their self identity. Both friend and foe are still an other. Their foundation for the true experience of full Awareness will always be shaky.

We now move on to inherited limitations and identities. Acquired identities and limitations are an individual effort. They stem from choice by one who has the autonomy to do so. Inherited limitations and identities are the result of group think and effort. Family, culture, political, ethnic and social circles instill limitations and identities in the minds and hearts of those less able to decide for themselves. Those who rely on a group for their psychological, emotional, physical, spiritual or economic support are particularly vulnerable to this inheritance.

Other influential group pressure may be gender-centered, religious or from government leadership. At the level of inherited limitations and identities, the illusion of a self is amplified and compounded. This fact also makes this expression of self-and-other exponentially more pervasive, constricting and difficult to transcend. Once this self-making becomes a group phenomenon some decisions must be made. These decisions include (1) what things will be named/labeled as and (2) who is in charge of naming them. Examples: What is "justice?" What is "freedom?" What is "healthy or unhealthy?" What is "meaningful?" What is "success?" Which group is "superior?" What is "Truth?" Who is "God?"

Some of those names will be seemingly innocuous while others will be intentionally mean-spirited, inflammatory and hurtful. We can now see how self-and-other literally gives birth to a hydra. For as many false distinctions you make based on self-and-other the more naming and creation of other-others becomes necessary. One interesting thing to note about this process is that as it grows eventually your false self begins to feel overwhelmed and lost among the myriad others it has created in the mind.

The outcome of the aforementioned activity creates yet another level of deception involved in self-making. All communication now becomes tainted because of the artificial difference created by self-making. How so? Disharmony and obstruction now have a home in the flow of your mind.

In order to establish an appearance of organization, a way of expressing or articulating differences must now be constructed. This is how the emergence of the phenomenon called *language* came into being along with its taxonomy of life and beings.

The second outcome of disharmony and obstruction having a home in the flow of your mind is that duality arises as a phenomenon. Now that the duality of self-and-other is created in the mind any articulation by a self will necessarily be dualistic. How else is it to maintain the facade of separateness? The moment this duality becomes the blurred lens through which life is experienced, other essential phenomena conducive to peace, unity and compassion likewise become fragmented and distorted.

Within the false appearances created by a self-and-other orientation, there is a gravitational pull down to lower states of consciousness. These lower states of consciousness perpetuate the illusion of separateness. On this lower level of vibration, the willingness and ability to experience existence as whole, rather than many separate parts, is obstructed. This is the fall from harmony into disharmony…from unity into a false multiplicity…from compassion to depraved and conscious indifference.

What we've stated so far, when directed toward any phenomenon you view as separate or other-than-your-self, immediately exposes how bias and discrimination emerge. Further, it shows you the roots of your unconscious behavior. It is your belief in (via word, action and thought) duality and a false sense of a self that allows you to persist in ignorance, or cruelty and abuse of the manufactured other. This you are able to do even though actual facts to the contrary of the false notions held by your-self are presented.

What are some of the behaviors your-self engages in that harm the whole? It is highly unlikely that a single day goes by that your-self does not engage in activities, big or small, that negatively impact this self and the others it has created. Any clinging to a notion of a self is like an immune system that has turned against the body. That which is actually suppose to protect the whole from harm (i.e. disease) is now experienced as the cause of harm. Please reflect upon this deeply.

The false sense of duality is undoubtedly supported by your-self's attachment to sensory data. Sensory data is all phenomena presented through sight, touch, taste, smell, thought and sound. Taken individually, each sense presents only a fragment of reality. That is, if you had no other sense other than sight you would think the only reality is form. If the only sense you had was hearing, you would think reality consisted only of sound. Do you understand this? But, for a being experiencing all six senses at once, reality appears to be fragmented and multiple. This is because of the rapidity and frequency at which sense data is presented and recycled.

For example, if you routinely unconsciously consume something, though it may be harmful, you'll continue to do that simply because your-self likes or wants it. Your-self, what it likes and the harm it creates have nothing to do with each other. In your mind, these are all separate and unrelated. The sense of a self combined with the duality created by it naturally leads to irrational non-compassionate speech, thoughts and actions. The act of otherizing is nearly unconscious when your-self has taken over. The longer this falsehood persists the more that otherizing becomes a conscious activity.

You do harm knowingly but then attempt to rationalize and justify it based on the notion that "that other is not me." This is how slavery became possible, the abuse of women became acceptable and the consumption of sentient-beings became, and presently remains, morally and ethically agreeable for many. Once one has been slave long enough to the self they've created, even when the gate of freedom opens up, the slave will often consciously remain in chains out of fear of complete freedom.

The addiction to a notion of self is the most pervasive addiction in the human realm. I firmly believe that addiction of any sort begins not with biology or chemistry but rather with the false reality created by the self. This is apparent when it comes to food and nutritional choices. It has been said that a dog will not bite the hand of its master. Why? Simply because it would not be wise to bite the hand that feeds it.

Under the influence of your-self you routinely bite your own hand. Sometimes that pain is experienced directly. However, often it may not be immediately experienced directly due to your-self's otherizing. Consuming sentient beings (or things extracted from them), destroying nature for profit and similar activities don't register as "pain" because your-self is not whole. These are not activities of a fully Aware being but rather one absorbed in selfhood. The more one recognizes the false appearance of self-and-other (i.e. duality) the more one begins to "feel the pain" of biting one's own hand (i.e. a lack of separation) and deep shifts in consciousness begin to happen.

When I first encountered this notion of no-self many years ago it was quite difficult for me to embrace. As a young spiritual seeker I was eager to free myself from entrapments of life that I viewed most people, including myself, to be unnaturally shackled to. Though I had made many improvements like becoming conscious about what I ate, I still felt a sense of being "caught in the game." To believe I had no self, literally not figuratively, seemed like a state of consciousness that was impossible for me to experience. My first breakthrough did not happen until I ceased resisting this possibility and began to reason and live from this "place" as though it were true.

The thought of literally not having or being a self was honestly frightening to me. I had grown up in a culture (i.e. United States) that teaches self glorification and ego-centric worship. To express one's self-hood and individuality is considered essential to being healthy and more successful in life. In this culture celebrities, entertainers and virtually anyone who appears regularly on television, or the in the media, is held on a pedestal. A person could be utterly belligerent and bellicose, but if that behavior could sell tickets or generate revenue it is more than ok…it is financially and socially rewarded.

Given my mental and societal baggage, I felt that embracing any notion of a non-self would not only mean less economic success but that I might in fact lose my mind. It is the latter concern that scared me the most. I thought there is no way a person can remain sane without self-identity. No way! How could I function in the world without preserving the only thing that I was absolutely certain of…that is that I am me. This body, this mind and these thoughts are uniquely my possessions. I could not consciously dispossess these even if I tried.

I grappled for nearly 10 years in silence with this no-self notion. This was calling into question everything I was taught and believed. Whether religiously, or academically, this concept just did not fit. How would I relate to other people if I went down this path? They would think that I was crazy. If I don't have a self then what does all of this mean? What are we doing here? I thought that life would feel so impersonal, hollow and cold without a subjective self to experience it.

Though I had so many fears about this no-self existence, I could not stop thinking about it or meditating on it. I had read so many writings and books about eastern sages, saints, gurus and mystics who appeared to have lived this way. They seemed to have completely different responses to the kinds of situations that we all find ourselves in life. From people dying, severe illnesses and many other versions of suffering, I saw that they had something (or perhaps lacked something) that allowed them not to suffer. There was one sense of this non-self consciousness that allowed me to semi-relate to all of this.

I have been a life long martial artist since age 11. I was introduced to meditation at that young age. I even had set up a home-made meditation alter. I imagine my mother thought it was strange but thankfully she only asked me a few questions about it and did not prohibit me from making it. I was born and raised in the Southern Baptist tradition. So, my meditation practice, along with the photos and adornments, would have been viewed as absolutely strange and likely idolatrous.

My meditation alter was made out of a plastic crate that was used for carrying bottles of milk. I turned it upside-down and placed a large bath towel over it. On top, I put a few photos of some martial arts masters I deeply admired as well as some fresh flower pedals, incense, candles, a burner and some martial arts books. I had a white bandana with the yin-yang sign on it that I would tie on my head each time I meditated. What a site that must have been for an 11 year old!

As I would kneel down, close my eyes and meditate I felt such a calm. But, admittedly it also felt strange. It felt strange because I would think why do I feel so calm when I'm not doing anything? I would think to myself you are just sitting and breathing. I figured this was all that was necessary as the masters on television did it the same way. Likewise, before and after each karate class we knelt down to meditate. It was through these formative years of meditation practice that I got my first sense of no self. However, I did not have the vocabulary to describe it as such at that young age.

My meditation practice coupled with the consistent intense martial arts training is where I was able to consciously experience the non-self. Yet, it was not an effortless continuous flow of this non-self consciousness. I could "get myself into the state" for a purpose but once that time had passed so went that state of consciousness. I'll give you a couple of examples. In my martial arts training we were required to go beyond the physical limitations of the body. Back in those days, there were only two divisions of classes. Twelve and under students were in one class and 13 and older students were in the adult classes. Further subdivisions were made by belt ranks within these two age categories.

Being 10-12 years old one felt like king or queen of the mountain. That is you were stronger, had better coordination and more skill than the younger students in your classes. But, when you were 13-15 in class with fully grown adults it was a different story. I recall one night during sparring when I was 13, I had my nose bloodied by a man who had to be at least 21 or 22 years old. It was a front kick to the nose. I had on a white gi (i.e. karate practice uniform) and the top of it had blood splattered all over it.

My instructor stopped the match and was visibly upset with the other student. My instructor accompanied me to the bathroom. My eyes were glossy which often comes with a bloody nose. I was grabbing paper towels and dowsing them with cold water as I held back my head and applied pressure to my nose to stop the bleeding. I caught a glimpse of my instructor in the mirror and he asked me, "what do you want to do?" I was not sure what he was asking me. After a momentary pause, still looking in the mirror at him standing behind me, I said " I want to fight." He stared at me for a moment and then slowly nodded his head agreeing to allow me to continue.

Apparently, my instructor had issued some push-ups to the other student. The standard penalty push-ups for showing lack of physical, mental or emotional control was 50. This person was very arrogant. As we resumed the match he had a smirk on his face as if to say "still have not learned your lesson?" All I wanted was to land one really good blow. I stepped out of my fear, my pain and anger to focus everything I had on landing that one strike. I knew that he would come charging in on a straight line to try to finish me.

When he came charging in I stepped off of that straight line and executed a spinning back-fist which landed square on his jaw. It knocked out one of his teeth. The match was stopped there. I had that scar on my knuckles for many years. It would serve as a reminder of my first conscious experience of what we call *mushin* (i.e. no mind) in karate. I would go on to have many more experiences of mushin during my training. This included belt ranking exams that lasted five to seven hours. These tests included full contact takedowns executed out in the parking lot, running, drills and calisthenics until people literally passed out and collapsed. After all of this, we had to spar.

This experience of *mushin* was the closest experience in my awareness that I could associate with non-self. I had to rely on it more times than I can count. Surprisingly, this experience also helped me in many other aspects of my life, including academic and professional. I found that my ability to consciously not merely "think outside of the box" but rather "step out of the box" was incredibly valuable and useful. Throughout my life I have been seen as unshakable and hard to rattle. This is because I actually practiced *mushin* in the dojo, professionally and in other real life situations.

I strongly believe that but for my experience of *mushin* that the experience of non-self would have remained entirely inaccessible to me. Furthermore, as valuable as *mushin* was and is, it did not seem as all-encompassing as the experience of no-self that I was exploring. Perhaps they are precisely the same and it was only my attachment to a concept expressed under particular circumstances that created a barrier to me believing non-selfhood could be possible. But, it did open the door to a conscious experience of going beyond the mind, emotions and biology and still being able to act.

Like my martial arts training, my spiritual journey was one where I was not interested in lofty ideas. I was not interested in having "spiritual experiences" or chasing moments of wonder. I was a seeker, who contrary to popular sentiments, believed that the answers were more important than the questions. The perpetual investigation of questions did not interest me though I spent decades investing and looking into many spiritual ideas, concepts, traditions and practices. It's been said that experience is the best teacher. I believe this is true. I'll briefly explain how this played out in my first **full** direct experience of non-self.

I had fallen on really hard times. Lost my business, all of my money and frankly my confidence. It did not matter to me that thousands, if not millions of other people were going through the same thing at that time. I was accustomed to powering through, making a way out of no way. I had overcome tremendous challenges and had always landed on my feet. This time was different. My understanding and application of *mushin* seemed not to be working. I could not understand why it was not working. I reached a point of being flat broke and sleeping in my car…for a long time.

I can't begin to innumerate the levels of depression, anxiety and borderline insanity (literally) that I experienced. The situation I was in was not real to me. I felt I was living some stranger's life. This could not be me. A homeless distraught soul starving, cold, alone and living in his car? All I could think of is how I had graduated college, always made good money, lived in wonderful places and have consciously tried to be kind to others. What I didn't realize was that the exploration and grappling with the non-self experience was unfolding within me.

Sometimes I would spend 8-10 hours in my car at a time because I had no where to go. I did not sleep well at night because I am a light sleeper and every noise would wake me up. Likewise, sitting upright all night (it was a 2 seater car with little room to recline the chair) and trying to sleep was nearly impossible. It was the worst state I had ever been in. I reached a point where I could no longer even think about it. Days would pass by in a blur. I could hardly re-member what happened just moments before due to malnu-trition and lack of sleep.

On one particular day I managed to have my "meal of the day" around mid-morning. It was a cup of tap water with a teaspoon of honey swished around in it. Many days that was all I had to eat. But, on this day it was all coming to a plateau of pain. I went back to my car and parked in an un-derground parking lot. By this time, it had been nearly 11 months of this unbelievable pain and suffering. I had no tears, no words and no thoughts left to analyze my situation or even grieve. I had exhausted all means of trying to main-tain my-self.

This day, I was slumped over the steering will. My stomach was growling so loud it was hurting my ears. Then the spinning started. I closed my eyes hoping not to fall over. It didn't work. Somehow I how fell sideways over the center console and was too weak to pull myself up. The spinning increased at such a rate that I can't presently articulate as it would not do it justice. I stayed in this position from morn-ing until just before sunset. During this time, I felt myself going into deeper and deeper levels of what I believed was death. Oddly, I use to refer to my car in those days as my coffin. I was sure I was going to die in this car…and I did.

I'd like to share a few things I remember about this particular death. I don't remember most of it. This is not because I have forgotten. I was fully aware the whole time. But, had no particular content or point of focus. I was just here. No coordinates. As the spinning continued, I started to see a bunch of colors swirling around in one big whirlpool. But, it was not dark. It seemed like a swirl of feint beige and bright light.

Initially, it seemed as though I was falling into it. But then it seemed like I was floating up into. Then it appeared I was floating side-to-side and back and forth in it all at once. What I mean to say is I lost complete contact with my body, my mind and everything else. It was terrifying because it was an experience devoid of bounds. As I write this, I feel I am not able to explain it. All I know is I was sure this was the end and that I was forever going into some other state which was death.

I had no thoughts…yet was fully aware. Not of my body, thoughts or anything else physical. I just knew that *something* was present. That something was present that could not experience anything. That is, it could not be touched, moved, manipulated or articulated as I am presently trying to do. I thought I had passed out, but after several hours of this the senses started to return.

First, I felt the stomach pains and heard the growling once again. Next the soreness in my right ribs because of the gear shifter in the center console being lodged there for hours on end. I felt like I had been clubbed in the head but there was no pain. I was waiting to open my eyes to see what was happening to me. I suddenly realized my eyes were open but I was still seeing that swirl!

I kept blinking my eyes. After a few moments the only thing I could see was the floor mat on the passenger side because my face was pressed to it. I thought I had already sat up when in actuality I was still slumped over the center console. My head was on the floor and my feet were up against the driver side window partially lodged between it and the steering wheel. I saw what appeared to be drool on the passenger side mat. I felt really groggy, still extremely hungry but surprisingly alert. More alert and aware than I had ever been in my life. I let my head fall back on the seat not trying to understand what happened to me because I already knew. I had crossed over…

Everything I had read and explored about the non-self had experientially become reality. In a flash, the thousands of pages read, innumerable conversations, prayers, fasting, meditation and training came and went. From that point until now I've had no more questions. What I mean is that I had no more questions about spiritual matters. All of the apparent differences in religious and spiritual practices and philosophies were consolidated into one experiential knowing. My silent mantra which I have not shared publicly until now was simply "only This." Later it simply became "…" (silence)

Part of the reason I was homeless so long is because I was committed to knowing the truth no matter the cost. Don't misunderstand me. I did not want to be there. I just embraced the now as is. I prayed out loud saying that "whatever I must endure or experience to know Truth directly…let it happen to me." The prayer was painfully answered. What I know is that the self is not real but rather a conditional experience. Beyond starvation, loneliness, self-pity and pain it cannot exist. Beyond emotions, mind, concepts and attachments a self cannot exist. Self-hood can be consciously transcended.

The Buddha is reported to have said the second most valuable gift you can give another is the gift of fearlessness. I finally understood true fearlessness. As a martial artist, a professional and a self I had thought fearlessness had to do with boldness, ferocity, grit and courage. It has nothing to do with any of these things. It is the lack of attachment to outcome and phenomena. Once self-hood has been annihilated these other self created illusions die with it. They are not consciously removed but rather just fall off as there is no-self there to host them.

As investment in self-identity and the illusion of duality begins to diminish, and eventually is eliminated, your mind settles into a state of equanimity and ease. You are no longer constantly trying to manage the illusion of otherness and can see the interdependence of all phenomena clearly. Likewise, it is in this state of consciousness that your capacity for compassion increases immensely without effort. You realize that everything you say, do, think…and eat has impact on the whole. Though your senses, and people around you, will continue to present existence as many separate pieces you will be able to function within that paradigm without suffering.

I ask you at this point in our contemplation to pause and reflect on the following questions. These questions should be deeply explored, one at a time, until you arrive at a clear experiential (non-intellectual) answer. Ponder these questions in light of what has just been presented to you so far.

1. If I were not under the veil self-identity, how would that impact my eating habits?

2. What levels of consciousness might be accessible to me minus my attachment to a self?

3. From *where* would I act, and make decisions, if not from a self-centered "I"?

4. With whom, or what, could I express more compassion with that I'm presently unable to because of self-identity?

You can't be considered a good manager when you're not fully aware of what it is you're actually managing.

~Sensei

If you are like most people, you likely refer to a particular biological phenomenon as "my body." How well do you manage this body? What do you really know about it besides that it gets hungry, tired, has desires, lives and dies? The fact is today most people are more likely to know more about the details of a celebrity's life, the season statistics of their favorite sports team or the lyrics to a popular song than they do about this body they claim to own. Is this you?

There is a level at which the biological experience in Consciousness goes undetected or unnoticed by the senses. While you are preoccupied with myriad thoughts and activities there is a world "within a world" that relies upon your management. This world is literally right beneath your nose, in your nose, beneath and above the skin surface and in your gut. Your lack of awareness of this world is a good indication of your management of it.

If you are able to maintain the meditative concentration created by the first chapter then this chapter's contemplation will enhance that experience. The purpose of the present contemplation is to demonstrate that reliance purely upon the senses (i.e. sight, taste, smell, feeling, hearing and thought) is not enough for you to fully comprehend the nature of the biological experience you call "my body." In fact, sole reliance on the senses can create a barrier to fully understanding the body.

Sense data presents the world to your awareness only as parts. For example, if you had no other biological sense data except for sight you would think the world consists only of forms. Furthermore, you would not even be able to detect the world that we will explore in this contemplation called the human microbiome. Likewise, the same would be true of sound. If you only had the sense of hearing you would think the world consists only of sounds. This would play out the same way for all of the others senses considered in the same way.

Due to technological advances, instruments have been created that allow us to see into the previously unseen world of the human microbiome. To say that this is literally a world within a world is no overstatement. A proper understanding of this biological phenomenon will help you realize that the human body itself is an ecosystem. Your awareness, serves as its manager. Let's take a closer look at what this world consists of to discover its direct relevance to our present contemplation.

The human microbiome contains 10 times as many cells from microorganisms as it does it does from human cells. To put this staggering number into perspective, today scientist estimate that the human body has about 37 trillion human cells. The human microbiome consists of viruses, bacteria, fungi and protozoa. These all live in and on the human body. These are all living entities. Each of them require a particular environment and sustenance to function properly.

Microbes can serve many functions. They may digest food to help generate nutrients for host cells and detoxify carcinogens. Microbes also activate and support the immune system as well as help digest fiber. They serve several other functions as well. Interestingly, there is no single microbe that is present in all parts of a single human body nor one common to all human bodies.

There is a mind boggling degree of bio diversity within the human microbiome. Generally speaking, greater levels of microbial diversity are associated with overall greater health of the body. For example, it is common that people with low microbial diversity in their guts are much more prone to obesity, Crohn's disease and inflammatory bowel disease. The number of genes in all of the microbes in one person's microbiome is 200 times the number of genes in the human genome.

So what is the origin of microbes? They are acquired during the birth process from the mother. As the physical being passes through the birth canal it essentially receives a "microbial bath." This level of interconnectedness and interdependence involved here should further divest any notion of selfhood or complete individuality. The human body is literally teeming with multiple habitats and life forms. All of this activity is happening simultaneously at every moment yet undetected by the senses.

"Know thyself" is a profound wisdom that has come down through the ages. Here we are taking this wisdom to another level of profundity. Claiming to be a self, or to have a self, is a frivolous and futile endeavor given the immensity of what we have just shared. The human body has infinitely more complexity, diversity and nuances of which you are likely completely unaware.

What it would take for you to truly know the human body in its entirety is beyond your capabilities based on what you presently call your-self. That is why it is absolutely imprudent to cling to the limited aspects of body you are more aware of and make major decisions (like what to eat) based upon such skewed and limited knowledge. Is awareness of physical appearance, unfettered subjective desires, fatigue and hunger really enough to say that you know this biological phenomenon you call **your** self? No, it is not. There is an alternative approach.

Here we have introduced only one of the many fascinating facts about the human body. You need not fully understand the "science" of it for our purposes. What is most important is that you begin to experientially verify the truth of interdependence. The human body itself is an amalgamation of numerous living ecosystems. Every region of the body somehow coalescing, or not in the case of illness or disease, with each other based upon decisions you make regarding several factors. The food you consume is one of those key factors.

To the naked eye, none of what we have discussed here can be seen. It is because of this most people make decisions about what they eat that ultimately cause them and other beings to suffer. You are responsible for managing multiple worlds and trillions of bio beings with every morsel of food you eat. Here is a difficult question you must ask yourself. The human body is a living multi-world. How good of a manager of these bio-worlds are you? Fortunately, you don't have to guess.

You can know how good of a manager you are in many simple ways. Look in a mirror. What do you see? If you are able to walk, try walking up and down one flight of stairs. How is your breathing after doing this? How many medications are you presently on or are likely going to need? Why do you need them? How many of your friends, family members or colleagues have cancer, diabetes, high blood pressure, hypertension or have died from any of them? What were their eating habits? Do their choices resemble yours? If so, you should expect the same outcome for yourself or worse.

Complete reliance on sense data will not allow you to discover the fullness of what is present. What is presented to the human senses is by no means illusory but extremely limited. It should be clear to you now that continuing to make decisions about what you eat based upon such limited information inevitably results in harm. Though you are not able to see this multi-world you are managing you are able to feel the effects of it. Unfortunately, the effects most often experienced are associated with mismanagement. Pain, lethargy, disease, anxiety, depression, stress and frequent colds are all signs of mismanagement and neglect due to lack of awareness.

Let's now contemplate the fullness of what is present in our awareness as it relates to body. You need to feel into what is not apparent to the senses. This seemingly finite body needs to be understood as multiple-worlds with innumerable bio-beings which have specific needs and requirements. How in tune are you with these worlds and the bio-beings that live there. If you have little to no idea about the interdependence and complexity of the biology you are presently experiencing, how can you legitimately claim ownership of it? Why would you chose to identity as it?

The point here is not that you need to be a physician or should have the knowledge of a scientist about human biology. Rather, what should be clear now is that (1) your senses can only grasp a tiny part of reality and (2) what you've been calling your-self does not even account for the totality of what's present in this assertion. Can you reasonably claim to be what you don't know exists? No, you cannot.

One should not fall into the mistake of shifting identity from that which the senses are aware of to that which they are not. To do so would be to merely trade one false identity for another. Here we are proposing something far more radical. You must not self identify with the body or any particular part of it. Let's use a hypothetical situation to enhance our contemplation. There is a person who has owned a car for 5 years and wants to sell it to you. You are interested but have a list of questions. If that person answered 95% of your questions with the response "I don't know" would you buy that car? You: Has this car ever been in an accident?

Seller: I don't know

You: When was the last time it had any repairs?

Seller: I don't know, but it has a great sound system

The above hypothetical seems absurd. You should note that this is likely how you would sound if one with knowledge were to inquire with you about this biology you claim to be. Other than physical characteristics (e.g. color of your hair etc), things you may be allergic to, likes and dislikes, your knowledge about the body is probably like the seller of the car. You're attached to the body, completely identify as it and have a surface level understanding of what's present.

Our brief contemplation about the human microbiome is intended only to illustrate one of many phenomena that you may be completely unaware of but are having a direct impact upon through your eating habits. If you are completely unaware of this biodiversity right under your nose, in your body and on your skin then how aware could you possibly be about the earth and your eating habits impact on it? Furthermore, what beings that your senses do detect are being harmed due to your eating habits and fixation on body-as-the-self?

Do you find it noncontradictory to eat a chicken, or other animals, but are repulsed at the thought of throwing your family pet into your oven? If so, there is one primary factor that accounts for this. You have a relationship with your pet that you don't have with other similar sentient beings. Note however that your sensory data as it relates to your compassion for life is limited only to the lives in your immediate sensory field. Your-self and your pet.

The sentient being in your immediate awareness, presence or living space is an animal that is treated like a family member. The sentient beings you purchase to eat are simply "meat" to be consumed for your pleasure and to satiate your hunger. Your present level of awareness, coupled with your identity as the body, has severely limited the extent of your understanding of interconnectedness. Likewise, these two factors contribute greatly to misunderstandings about the negative impact of your eating habits and choices on the micro and macro levels of existence. The self's habit of otherizing simply classifies the pet as friendly-other and other animals as food-other. Hence, the difference in your treatment, compassion and concern. It's not because you're "a bad person."

Let's take up another intriguing phenomenon of body of which you may not be aware. The human electromagnetic field. For thousands of years, many spiritual traditions, primarily eastern or indigenous, have taught about the human aura. It's a deeply spiritual phenomenon that is observable by those devoid of self-identity. There is a great deal of instruction and teachings on what this aura is. Depending on the tradition, it may be referred to as aura, chi, astral body, bliss body or perhaps the soul. For the purposes of this contemplation, we will use the western scientific term of *electromagnetic field*.

The human electromagnetic field (hereafter HEF) is not believed to be perceptible by the human senses. This is the view according to western science. This is not a belief strictly held in many indigenous or eastern spiritual traditions. In any case, the first matter to be addressed is what is the HEF? How does it work? These are interesting questions. Entire books and studies have been written about them. For the present purpose of this contemplation, it is only necessary to understand the HEF on a conceptual level.

The HEF is essentially the human body's energy field. This field is created by billions of electrical charges throughout the body. These electrical charges are essential for the healthy functioning of the trillions of cells in the body. Each cell is conducting approximately 7,000 actions per second. That is an astonishing amount of activity. Without electrical charges this activity could not take place.

Cell membranes serve as the mangers and facilitators of electrical charges. Though the voltage level of each cell is quite low in comparison to a house appliance, collectively it it plays an important role in keeping the human body moving. Not only does each cell have its own electromagnetic field, but so does each organ. The sum of these is what is meant by the HEF. The cellular membrane level process involved with optimizing and managing the health of the cell itself creates the electrical charge.

Similar to the human microbiome, the HEF is not observable by the senses but is directly impacted by the food one consumes. A lack of the awareness of the HEF's existence and purpose on a purely biological level is a major shortcoming. The strength and vibrancy of this field is deeply impacted by your food choices and eating habits. This should be easy to deduce even with this simple explanation of the HEF and its processes. When voltage levels cease to be sufficiently maintained in enough cells the human body experiences dis-ease and will ultimately cease all activity.

It is worth pondering how is it that various spiritual traditions were able to detect this field of energy without modern tools and technology. Perhaps it's not as strange as it may first appear. It's likely that you have thought that someone's presence (i.e. aura or energy field) was particularly pleasant, distinct or odd. That person may not have said a single word to you or have made any contact with you. But, somehow you just "felt something." This experience is simply the meeting of two energy fields. The strength, weakness and breadth of each respective field produces a unique co-field experience. It could be one of attraction, repulsion or confusion.

Whether you think of the HEF and human microbiome individually, or together, they exemplify just how much is happening in the body beyond sensory observation. It is fair to say that you truly know very little about the body you are presently experiencing. Yet, the urge to identify with and as a body remains so strong. What purpose does this serve? Not one that is beneficial. It is simply a habit that can be broken with intention.

Self-identifying with the observable parts of the body in fact limits the fullness of the experience of body. Expanding one's awareness about the whole has the opposite effect. Having become aware of the incalculable nuisances of the body one refuses to be shackled by any part of it. When the shackles of body identity are broken deeper states of consciousness, possibility and choice become available. Imagine what would be possible for you if you were not limited to what sensory data presents.

The experience of body is an intriguing one. You need not denigrate it. Likewise, you must not assign to it any special status simply because the experience of it seems so intimate and exclusive. The dominant preoccupation with the experience of body is solely due to your present inability to simultaneously direct your awareness to the broader field of phenomena. If you could ground yourself in the broader field in which the experience of body is merely a co-participant, the tendency to identify as body would significantly diminish. At deeper levels of consciousness, all identity as body ends.

CONTEMPLATION: Nature

Know the difference between world and earth.

~Sensei

The purpose of this chapter's contemplation is to continue to guide you out of the wilderness of the self you have constructed into a much deeper and vast state of awareness of interdependence and reality. If you have been paying close attention, and engaging with this text with focus, then the shackles of the self-centered "I" should be beginning to fall away. But there are likely still several challenges for you. One of these is the phenomenon called "nature." Let us now dispel the facade of the otherness of nature created by the self.

If you are like many people when you think of nature, what arises in your mind is what you believe to be an external phenomenon. You may imagine it as place where wild animals live. You may also think of beaches, rivers, mountains, forests or deserts and their respective weather patterns. Nature appears to have its own rules. Its forces also seem to be highly unpredictable if not unmanageable. From hurricanes, to earthquakes and fires, or animals with unbelievably superior strength and speed, the tendency is to have a like/fear relationship with nature.

Please pay very close attention to what follows next. We explored the senses and sensory data in the first contemplation. It is solely out of this sense data that you have created an I that does not exist. You'll recall that we discovered how

25

limited the senses are in presenting the fullness of existence. In fact, in the second contemplation we used the presence of the human microbiome to show how multiple ecosystems with billions of bio-beings are going completely unnoticed by the senses. From a place of non-self and detachment from false appearances we will discover deeper truths about nature.

Please ponder the following question. How do you know nature? Whatever your experience of nature is it's likely based exclusively on sensory data. You base what you know of nature off of what you see, hear, feel, smell, taste and think. Recall what we now know about the manufactured self, its need to otherize and the extreme limits of sensory data. If this same self, along with the senses, are completely oblivious to the fullness of the experience of body, how could it be any more accurate about nature?

The phenomenon called nature is awesome. It is powerful, beautiful and diverse. Similar to the human body it is an ecosystem with a seemingly incalculable number of bio-beings which includes humans. Let's put this in perspective. One teaspoon (a single gram) of rich soil has more bio-beings in it than there are people on the planet. This tiny sample of nature will contain as many as 1,800 different varieties of bio-beings. Bacteria, fungi and microbes among them. This should sound familiar to another phenomenon we contemplated.

Let's take this nature contemplation to the next level. Because the manufactured self measures nature through the senses, and the limitations of "I", nature appears to be immense. The one truth the manufactured self is aware of is how small it is. Juxtaposed to nature the self cowers in the corner. It knows it is no match for nature in any way. Yet, there is an undeniable attraction to nature. This is the cause of the like/fear relationship many have with nature.

When the false appearance of self is removed and re-
placed with naked awareness there is a dramatic shift in experience of nature. It does not lose its beauty nor its impres-
siveness. But, from the vantage point of naked awareness
nature is no longer experienced as other. It also no longer
appears larger than Consciousness. This is an extremely subtle and important movement. Let's apply this to several situations.

In the presence of a huge mountain, tall tree or vast ocean
one identified with a self feels *small*. In that smallness, a
sense of awe and or fear will be present depending upon the
circumstances. If you were out on the ocean on a ship about
to sink, or standing next to a huge tree about to fall, you'd
likely be afraid. But, if you were simply standing on the
seashore on a lovely sunny day admiring the waves you'd
likely feel a sense of peace. However, no matter which scenario above was your experience the difference in your response (like or fear) would be exclusively based upon a
body-I orientation.

What do you imagine your experience would be in any of
the previous scenarios if you were not attached to the self
you've created? Take a moment to consider this question.
Then ask the same question but in regards to your everyday
life. Heretofore, you have lived as a manufactured self relying on sensory data that is helpful but ultimately inadequate
for experiencing the whole of existence. Nature serves as
one of many phenomena to remind you that this self you've
created is too small. One shake of the earth, a single wind
gust that shakes the airplane, or the growl of a big dog and
this false self becomes riddled with fear.

Through naked awareness (Consciousness directed at a
specific phenomenon) nature is experienced in a completely
different manner. As beautiful, immense and perhaps even
dangerous as it may be, nature is not bigger than naked
awareness. It can't be. On the other hand, the senses are vir-

tually short-circuited trying to comprehend the totality of nature. If so much life exists in a single teaspoon of soil, how can one possibly ever even think of knowing the entirety of nature? It seems absurd. It is precisely in this absurdity that you can find your path to naked awareness and enlightenment.

Nature presents to us the opportunity to literally experience the beyond-the-self. From nearly every religious or spiritual tradition there are scores of stories of individuals reaching enlightenment, or having profound experiences, initiated in nature. These individuals experienced naked awareness. Those who are able to continue to live in this awareness we call prophets, fully realized or enlightened. Those who exemplify this wisdom in their character we call sages, saints, holy, masters or awakened.

Naked awareness does not suddenly appear from somewhere. It is an ongoing ever-present experience. It is co-present with every moment of consciousness. For those who are mired in the web of body-I consciousness, nature has the ability to remove this veil entirely or enough to give you a glimpse of this co-presence. This is not because nature possesses any unique special powers. It is because the manufactured self cannot maintain its dominance in the presence of naked awareness. Nature appears to have a unique way of revealing the co-presence of naked awareness. In actuality it is the absence of myriad sensory data experienced in daily life coupled with the stillness of nature that allows for naked awareness to expose the false appearance of a self.

The attachment to body-I, and sole reliance on sensory data, allows you to make deliberate unconscious decisions. Now is a good time to take note of how you manage the body and how you relate to nature. If you are like most people you'll be forced to admit something is wrong. This has nothing to do with whether you are a "good or bad person." It has only to do with your degree of awareness. It should be clear that any degree of attachment to a sense of self will always lead to a severely diminished level of awareness.

This severely diminished level of awareness leads to alienation from nature. It is what allows you to desensitize yourself to the relationship that you are in with nature. Some of you may be thinking "I like nature and I don't do anything intentionally to harm it." Have you closely examined your eating habits? Not just what you eat but also how you eat? How you cook and store your food. What kind of materials you use. How your eating habits may be contributing to manufacturing processes that are poisoning the planet and/or harming sentient beings? (including humans) How do your daily choices show that you even care about these matters? These are deeper questions that only one with naked awareness could raise.

Here's another question that's relevant to this chapter's contemplation. When you think of nature do you think of food as part of nature? Or have you somehow given it a unique category of simply "food?" Excluding pseudo-foods produced in laboratories and passed off as fit for human consumption, food should be understood not simply from nature but rather **as** nature itself in a particular formulation. For example, as a grain, fruit or vegetable. For the one who is aware, this goes into yet another level of understanding.

For those who see with naked awareness, they know not only that food is nature, but that they, food and nature are not separate…literally speaking. Let's take a moment to digest this last point. It may seem too far of a stretch if you are still clinging to body-I. Your manufactured self, along with its inadequate sense data, may not be able to breathe at this spiritual altitude. That is good. Let it die. Bury it today.

The above truth can be demonstrated by what we have already contemplated here coupled with the following example. Real fruit comes from the earth. Earth is a representative form of the phenomenon called nature. The same is true of fruit. Food and nature are in fact not separate but the same. What happens when an apple is consumed? That apple initiates a process called digestion. During digestion the apple literally merges with the body. It becomes the body.

At no point has that apple ceased to be other than what it is…nature. Not pre or post digestion. Components of this apple are completely assimilated **as** the body not *into the body*. What is not used is released from the body. We must pause here to reflect upon how the manufactured self, and sense data, preclude one from clearly seeing at this level of truth. The self interjects and asserts that there are three different things involved here. A me, an apple and nature. We are all different. Nature is not apple and both are outside of me. This same false scenario plays out in regards to all of nature if perceived through a self.

Nature is full of diverse bio-beings as evidenced by the single teaspoon of rich soil. You can observe many colors, shapes, objects and sizes thanks to the senses and the data they present. For this reason, we should not demean the senses or sense data. But, if you are to live in harmony as nature, not with it, you must be able to see through the false appearances that lead to harmful decisions about food choices and consumption. You must not cling to the body-I concept. Non-clinging will allow you to experientially verify that nature is not an *other*.

Nature presents many opportunities for us to shatter the illusion of self-hood. One of the more obvious examples is via weather and the changing of the seasons. Let's look at the three phenomena we call hot, warm and cold in regards the phenomenon of weather. At this moment, while you are reading this book, is it hot, warm or cold outside? Where I am it's presently raining hard yet quite hot and humid. Generally, one would associate rain with it being cold, if not cool outside.

We can ask if nature is hot? What is the weather like where you are at this moment? Suppose you are somewhere where it is snowing or raining or with very low temperatures. Is nature cold? Is nature hot and cold? What about the seasons? At this moment, it's spring in one place, summer in another, winter another and fall in another. Is nature any of these individually? Is nature all of them collectively?

For the one who is aware, and not chained to a false sense of a self, the answers to these questions about weather are obvious. What a magnificent assistant nature can be in dismantling the body-I trap. Take note that the questions as posed present several options and possibilities as answers. They present a singular option, an either/or option and an all of the above option. Depending on your level of awareness one of these three will resonant more with you.

If you have little awareness, you will state that nature is as you are presently experiencing it in your area. If it's cold outside you would answer "nature is cold." If you are more aware, you will likely answer nature is both what you are presently experiencing and what another is experiencing in another area. If you see yourself as most opened minded you may answer that nature is all weather patterns collectively. However, there is another layer to this.

The above options, under which the majority of people would likely respond, are all still responses trapped in the dualism created by a self. There is a fourth option that only naked awareness would recognize. That nature is none of these phenomena individually or collectively. Perhaps this is a bit perplexing. How could nature **not** be any of these individually or collectively? Excellent question. Respond to this question through naked awareness rather than a self. How did naked awareness respond? Once again, it should be easy to see how a sense of self, the dualism it always produces and exclusive reliance on sense data will always obstruct you from the deepest truths about nature.

I have had many profound experiences in nature that demonstrated duality is merely a fiction created by a manufactured self. One took place during a meditation sit I was doing at the beach. There was beautiful white sand, turquoise water and a light lovely breeze. The sun was not intense but just warm enough to feel a light caress of rays on the skin. After a few rounds of chanting, I began my meditation.

As a practitioner of Chan Buddhism, I rarely ever fully close my eyes in seated meditation. I usually direct my gaze on the floor several inches away from my crossed legs. My eyes are only half closed at most. On this occasion I was sitting on the sand. The conditions seemed like they could not be better for a good meditation. I don't like to time my meditation sits. I prefer to just sit until I naturally come out of them. That has been as short as 5 minutes and as long as over an hour.

At some point, I was beginning to come out of this meditation. Before fully doing so, for some reason I slowly raised up my left hand. I was just staring at it against the background of the deep blue sky and the few white cotton ball-like clouds. With eyes still at half-mast, and looking at my hand with fingers spread wide, it was as though I could see through my hand. Meaning, my hand, the sky, sun and clouds appeared to be completely merged into one.

I was so focused that while I was aware that my hand was up I did not feel like I was exerting any energy whatsoever to hold my hand up. Furthermore, I could no longer feel any sensation of sitting on the sand. It was all so ethereal. That said, I did not feel I was in another realm or having an out of body experience.

This was not the only time that I've had such a profound experience of reality. I have experientially known for quite some time that duality and separation are illusions stemming from a false self and sense data. In fact, for years I have experienced this body as simply another phenomenon in which naked awareness had taken a particular interest in for many years. Ultimately, this body became too small to hold the attention of my awareness. It became neither an object of unnecessary obsession nor one to be abandoned. It's simply here in Consciousness like all other phenomena.

Long gone is the sense of a self looking out at the world. Literally no inside and outside while still fully cognizant of causes, conditions and effects as they relate to body. One formulation of these three can produce the phenomena of pain or tears. Another formulation can produce happiness. No matter what is produced I know I am not what I experience. I also know that these experiences all arise and fall yet something remains present and unchanged at every moment.

The experience on the beach was simply another beautiful moment of Truth. I shared this with you to illustrate that once you truly abandon the self, your moment-to-moment experience in life will leave no room for doubt about the absence of any separation from nature. The desire for proof, or chasing *spiritual experiences*, will abruptly end once the self falls away. The point is you are not nature and you are not not nature. Duality of any sort is a fiction. Once you experience the truth of this you'll experience no difference between nature and your awareness. This **will** lead to more conscious choices in your eating habits and practices.

Nature will still appear to be separate pieces only because that's how the senses and their data present all phenomena. However, the naked awareness will see through this illusion. Naked awareness can engage in the play of duality without suffering from it. Vibrant colors, different shapes, sizes and sounds will all continue to present themselves but a deeper wisdom will erase the false appearance of separateness. An enlightened being does not cease to experience what sense data presents, but is able to put that information into its proper context.

The cause of harmful eating choices is due to the belief in being a self. Naked awareness severely challenges the self with a deeper inner-knowing and lack of separation from nature. You become a full participant in the phenomenon called nature. This participation allows you to experientially verify the interdependence of all phenomena. There are no cultural arguments, ideological points of view or political allegiances involved at this level of awareness. Those are all concepts and diversions for people still blinded by self-hood.

We will now engage in an experiment. This experiment is meant to immediately get you into a deeper state of consciousness. Sit down somewhere in a comfortable position. If you can go outside please do. If you can do this at a park, beach, on a trail or anywhere else in nature it will be really helpful. Otherwise, simply sit near an open window or step outside your home or office to conduct this experiment.

Next, close your eyes. Take 3-5 deep breaths then let go of any sense of eye-sight. After another 3-5 deep breaths do the same regarding any sense of taste. Continue on with this process for the sense of smell and feeling. Allow only the sense of hearing to remain. Try as best as you can to focus your awareness exclusively on the sense of hearing. Once you feel you are focused only on the sense of hearing, take 15-20 slow deep breaths. Please take your time with this experiment. It should take you between 15-25 minutes to complete.

When the world is presented exclusively as sound what happens to your awareness? Does it decrease? Does it disappear? Does it deepen? What was your experience? Depending on your ability to engage in naked awareness, and focus without the mind wandering, you should experience less attachment. That is, when there is less sensory data the mind has fewer phenomena on which to cling.

You may have also noted that the sense of hearing was magnified. The longer you sat in this state, the more subtle sounds you seemed to be able to detect. This is the emergence of naked awareness which is co-present at every moment of consciousness. This is a great practice to facilitate experiential verification of a deeper state of consciousness that is ever available to you. Regularly practice this and alternate the sense that remains. Sometimes only sight or only feeling while the others are turned off. Ultimately, work your way up to turning off all of the senses at once… including thought.

CONTEMPLATION 4: Universe

If some day you are able to see it all, name it all and describe it all will you have increased in wisdom?

~Sensei

Modern science has given us a peak into the universe in ways that boggle the mind. It seems that new discoveries are made on a regular basis. It's difficult to keep up with them all. As the fields of science, such as quantum physics, attempt to explain the universe from unique angles, so too are technological tools becoming more sophisticated. There seems to be no limit to what science can do. Yet, it is not the only way, nor the most efficient way, of knowing the universe.

Please reflect on the following question. What is the goal of scientific inquiry? So much effort, resources and human energy is put into this endeavor, but to what end? Is the goal merely to explain all phenomena? If it were able to do so, what do you think that what mean for you existentially and spiritually? Perhaps you would no longer have a need for spirituality. Maybe knowing the name of everything that exists and how it works (from a purely mechanistic view) would make you God?

Perhaps science is still in search of the holy grail or tree of life. Its experts may be hoping that they can someday unlock the mystery of life and death. Maybe they hope to be able to control it. Every age believes its science is the most advanced there has ever been. Yet, when we survey history,

36

and how advanced a society is based upon its scientific ingenuity it's all relative. Many scientist will state that science only studies "what is." That is, it has no interest in or time for things that *don't exist*.

Today, when you look at the most industrialized and technologically advanced countries, it does not appear that they are necessarily also the happiest. Certainly they enjoy conveniences that other societies may lack, but they also seem to suffer from higher levels of nihilism and despair. In countries that are more technologically advanced, there are more ways to contact other people but the connection value seems to have suffered. Is this *because* of science or technology? Not entirely so.

There are a few radical thoughts about the scientific enterprise that are worthy of reflection. These thoughts are not meant to demean science but rather to put it into context so you may maximize its value. First, the realm of science is limited to facts and investigation related to phenomena not wisdom. Second, science has made no "discoveries" and never will. Let's exam these two statements in connection with a spectacular event that occurs in the universe.

Have you ever heard of a supernova? It is an incredibly powerful and literally explosive event. There are several types of supernovae but we will limit ourselves to the one most commonly known to the general population. Science defines a supernova as the violent explosion of a star. Essentially the core of the star collapses inward and results in an immense explosion. That is why this type of supernova is called *core-collapse* supernova.

These massive stars are eight times larger than the sun in our system. That is incredibly large. This gigantic explosion occurs in the last phase of a star's life. In its last phase of life, it cools down. Once the outward pressure of the star is no longer in harmony with the inward pressure…

boom! Gravity finishes this process which only takes seconds. This is hard to imagine for an object that is 15 times larger than the earth. What remains after this process will be either nebula (a dense core of hot gas) or a black hole.

Science has described this process for us. The above is a condensed version of the explanation. For our purposes, just take with you that a supernova is a massive star that violently releases an unbelievable amount of force into the universe. Having explained the process, it's a perfectly fitting point for science to move on to the next thing. It has explained *the how* of this phenomenal process. You have the information and science has fulfilled its role. You have the observable facts nothing else is needed.

What would happen if one were to look at the phenomenon of a supernova from the spiritual eye of wisdom? Beyond raw data, is there a truth to be discovered in the supernova event that does not require an in-depth knowledge of any science? The answer is yes. Do you know the components of a star? What materials make up a star? Almost every element listed in the Periodic Table are the result of a star's life and death. Furthermore, many of the elements that are released into, and create, the actual universe after a supernova event are exactly the same elements found in the human body.

Some of the elements produced in a stars life and death are iron, copper, hydrogen, magnesium, nitrogen and oxygen. Additionally, they can produce sodium, phosphorous, potassium, sulfur, chlorine and carbon. Every one of these 12 elements (and more) produced by stars are found in the human body! The human body is an electrically charged mineral-based organic bio-form. The are 102 minerals that can be found in the human body. Oxygen accounts for approximately 61% of the human body mass followed by carbon (22%), hydrogen (10%) and nitrogen (2.5%). These alone account for about 95% of human body mass.

We can now consider the scientific understanding about supernovae, elements/minerals, formation of the universe and human life to two of the major themes in this book: false appearance of a self and duality. The phenomenon called *universe* is for most people even more mysterious, grand and unknown than nature. But, you must remember what wisdom has shown you so far. That this so-called mystery and separateness is all based on the limited observation of a manufactured self and its sense data. Even science, with its sophisticated tools, is merely relying on mechanisms that magnify the reach of human sense perceptions. It has done this with some marvelous results.

However, if some day you are able to see it all, name it all or describe it all will you have increased in wisdom or merely gathered a lot of information? Here is where the co-presence of the spiritual eye can take information and transform it into wisdom on how to live. Given what you have just read about the universe, how should it impact your eating habits? You should see that the fundamental differences between what you believe to be your-self and the universe are more perceived than real.

This contemplation on the universe should be igniting many thoughts for you regarding enlightened eating. Much of this will depend on how deeply you are making the connection between all perceived phenomena, the limits of sense data and this self you claim to be. Moreover, you should be fully aware that by clinging to your manufactured self you are truly missing out on the direct experience of something far more grand, expansive and stable. It should be clear how you have developed eating habits based upon clouded perceptions. But, that is changing now. You are starting to see through the illusions of separation and otherness.

The statement was made earlier in this contemplation that science does not *discover* anything. At first glance, this may seem to be a radically incorrect statement. Let's continue our discussion of the supernova in concert with this statement. Here we must transcend the limits of language to get to the wisdom. Debate about the definition of the word *discovery* would be a waste of time. As the self begins to fall away, your language and thoughts should become more precise.

If we think of the word *discover* in its general use, it's meant to indicate that something new was brought to your attention. As it regards the universe, scientist often speak of discovering new stars, galaxies and other phenomena. With each new discovery the excitement encourages further investigation into the universe. Note that this scientific way of discovery is still limited to merely enhancing some aspect of human sensory organs. For example, a telescope extends what the eye can see. Another gadget may allow scientists to hear decimals otherwise imperceptible to the human ear.

Interestingly, many of the sages and illuminates of spiritual traditions have made miraculous observations about the universe without any mechanical tools or technology. They often spoke of an infinite universe with more planets than can be counted. Likewise, they have gone a step further than modern science is willing to go. They spoke of there being innumerable beings of various sorts with physical or ethereal constitutions suitable for their particular realms. They achieved these insights mainly through prayer, meditation and deep observation of their own minds.

These saints and wise people made these observations thousands of years ago. The western world has only recently begun to understand and *verify through science* what have been settled matters for centuries among other people. So, we can now raise the question about the use of the word *discovery* in contemporary times and particularly within science. Is it legitimate to discover something that already exists? Can you really discover something that has existed for thousands, if not millions, of years in the universe? No.

Using discovery in the way that it is used in contemporary society is problematic on at least three levels. First, it inflates the sense of a self. Second, it often reinforces a sense of separateness and duality. Third, it can lead to abuse and an unnatural relationship with that which was *discovered*. These are strong statements. Let's take a look at them individually.

You need not look beyond human experience to verify these statements. Often when people claim to have discovered something they immediately seek to appropriate it into their manufactured self. This is particularly true if they believe there is some financial gain to be had or that it would solidify some desire to be acknowledged or remembered. Today, we see this hubris play out in many ways in relation to the universe. One example is how people can actually purchase a registration to name a star after themselves.

We have repeatedly seen how explorers, conquerors, colonizers and religious zealots have torn entire civilizations apart. Often these societies had been in existence longer than the so-called discoverers themselves. That one could claim to have discovered a land that has had hundreds, if not thousands, of years of history exemplifies the danger of selfhood. You will note that on this planet when people discover places they immediately want to name the landscapes, cities, towns and streets after themselves. This is all an attempt of the self to inflate itself and its perceived importance. Essentially, it wants to say look at what **I** found.

Devoid of an attachment to a self you would have no desire to appropriate the universe in part or whole. Rather, each *discovery* would be seen not as a new *other* but an expansion of naked awareness. In the case of a star, you would note the shared ancestry between the body and the universe.

To claim a planet, or name a star after yourself, would seem redundant. It would be like giving the fingers on your hand your personal name. This would be absurd.

The self often fears the other it creates. One way the self feels more secure about the other is to own it. I discovered this star or particle so it should be named after me. I discovered the cure to this disease so it should bare my name. I discovered this mathematical equation about the universe so it should be named after me. I discovered this land so it, its people and resources belong to me. Do you see the pattern? Do you see the problem? It's the self needing to inflate its importance and existence.

Stars have incredibly long lives. Depending on the mass of a star its lifespan can range between several million years to billions of years. These are not phenomena that humans can claim to discover no matter when they actually experience them for the first time. It is incumbent upon those with deeper consciousness to refrain from using and perpetuating the use of words that reify self-hood. Here we see the problems that can be caused when discovery is used by those attached to the self they've manufactured.

The current use of the word *discovery* also reinforces a sense of separateness and duality. Both of these are false. If you are attached to self-identity, almost everything you experience or encounter would technically be a discovery. But, for the one not attached to self-identity the encounter deepens realization. Each phenomenon in consciousness points to an undeniable interdependence. The realization is that one is many and many are one.

For those who are trapped in self-identity, one is one and many are many. They can't conceive that one is in fact many and many are one. Let's use the supernova as a way to see the truth of this in the universe. From a single star exploding the result is many. More stars, more galaxies, black holes as well as minerals and elements are created from this single event. As we noted earlier, even human life was made possible in part due to supernovae. With each phenomenon created by a supernova, each phenomenon becomes the cause for the birth of many others. Through naked awareness wisdom once again shows us something even deeper about supernovae. One is many and many is one.

So, new phenomena and experiences serve as reminders (should one "forget") of the interdependence of phenomena and beings. While the senses may present a phenomenon as exclusively singular or many, the naked awareness shows the full picture. It allows for the co-presence of awe and wonder while not reinforcing dualistic thinking or a sense of separateness.

The ability to see beyond the false appearance of newness allows for a different relationship and mindset to emerge. One that does not seek to merely extrapolate value from an other for selfish or unsustainable reasons. This is an important insight to understand. Much of the abuse of the earth, sentient beings (especially humans and animals) is based upon the notion of discovery. It fuels dangerous thoughts that have proven to be utterly destructive and a source of disharmony.

The self-centered version of discovery has resulted in the belief that whatever the self encounters for the first time previously had no purpose, function or use. Further, that if it had any purpose, that purpose must now yield to the self's desires. The owner-owned, slaveholder-slave and dominant-subordinate paradigms all are born of this phenomenon. A false hierarchy based upon ignorance and lack of awareness creates an environment ripe for violence and conflicts to arise. Human history is full of examples of this fact.

The universe immediately becomes less alien the moment you erase the perceived differences between it and the self you've created. The form of a star verses the form of the human body appear different from one another simply due to physical properties. But the "material" of both are the same as has been demonstrated. If a human being dies of old age its not unlike the process of a supernova. The phenomenon called human being arises due to other causes and conditions, abides for some time and ultimately *burns out of energy*.

The balance and harmony between exhaling and inhaling ceases and with that so does the phenomenon of body. The supernova comes into being due to other stars and materials. At some point, the balance of outward pressure and inward pressure can't be maintained. Once this occurs the form of that particular star ceases to exist. However, that so-called death simply merges with, and creates, more forms and life.

It is interesting to note how the concept of reincarnation is constantly displayed by the universe. The supernova is a prime example of this. While the body (or form) of the particular star ceases, the star's life-force does not. The manufactured self clings to forms via data presented by the eyes. Due to this clinging, it believes that only what it sees is the real thing or exists.

To the self, if a form is no longer perceptible by the eyes, then it no longer exists. Yet, in truth, the life-force continues by creating more forms. These forms are perceived to be *new* to the one attached to a self. In actuality, these forms are none other than the one that co-created them. Again, we see the wisdom and truth that one is many and many is one. If you begin to regularly gaze up into the universe, you will experience profound realizations about the interdependence of existence. You don't need a high powered telescope. Your naked awareness and eyesight are sufficient.

I have had several amazing experiences and awakenings while observing the sky. One late evening, I went out to the beach to look at the sky and stars. The stars that night seemed so bright that I felt I could reach out and touch them. Virtually no clouds were present in the sky. I had an unobstructed view. Stars are at a minimum several light years away from the earth. One light year is about 5.88 trillion miles. That is astonishing in and of itself. Presently, there is no technology that would allow a human being to physically travel to a star.

After about 20 minutes of staring at these beautiful bright bulbs in the sky, a thought came to me that lingered for a while. How is it that something could be trillions of miles away and this being can see it? One feels so insignificant and small compared to such an awesome phenomenon as a star. I began to think how difficult it is to make out the particular features of someone's face standing only 100 yards away, yet I can see a part of something light years away. It's actually quite amazing. How can this be?

When I raised this question I was not in search of a scientific answer. I was not asking for a calculation or theory to explain a physical experience. Rather, I was inquiring into the nature of reality itself. What could be the purpose of the human being possessing the ability to see deep into the universe with the naked eye? By this time, I was about 45 minutes into my star gazing. Then I had a wonderful opening.

After acknowledging experientially that I and that star are not separate, I wondered from where is this question arising? In questioning how I was able to see something far away, yet not something else much closer, I realized how subtle a sense of a self may try to lure one into dualistic questioning. I deeply observed how the senses persistently force questions steeped in a false otherness. I thought I was so small compared to such a huge phenomenon. The **only** reason I appeared different from that star was because of the sensory data (sight and thought) presented at the moment. An element of humor suddenly arose in me. Given the limits of sensory data, that star only appeared to be the size of a small button.

I thought I'd continue this cosmic play for a little while longer. I pondered "seeing" the current experience from the star's side. I thought how absurd to raise such a question. It was in this absurdity that I realized how one's mind can be impacted by the perceived presence or absence of sentience. I am able to experience this star and sentience simultaneously. I can choose to identity as the "smaller" of what is being presented to my present awareness. The smaller being the sentience of the human body. I could instead identity as the larger body of the star rather than the small human body. I could identify as both. But, I chose to neither identify nor not identify with either phenomena without conflict. Too many concepts involved. Bigger, smaller, sentient, non-sentient, far and near are all body-I concepts that can trap one in self-hood.

Acknowledging these attachment traps, made the question disappear. I realized that if I choose not to identify with the sentience of the human body, nor with the awesome stature of the star, that there was no conflict. The question became irrelevant. There was no sense that I was more or less. What remained was only an awareness of the illusion of duality. This experience was many years ago. I was not yet able to carry that wisdom in all circumstances. But, during the drive home, and the entire following day, I remained somewhat in a dream-like state about what I had learned from that star gazing experience.

Everything I experienced through the senses the following day made me realize how calculations and comparisons about phenomena are constantly happening. Some are quite conscious while others are not. I also realized that the more habitual these comparisons are the more unconscious

and subtle they become. Each time it happens the false appearance of self-hood is reinforced and becomes more difficult to detect. Since that powerful night whenever I look up into the cosmos I realize that I'm looking into a constituent phenomenon of something I'm already deeply familiar with which is this body. All phenomena are interdependent. Without one the other cannot exist. As a practical self-verifying practice, exam anything you've observed in the universe to see if in fact it has an independent existence. The ultimate truth will spring forth with such force you'll feel as though you have made a new *discovery*.

The differences between the power of the mind, selfhood and the body has nothing to do with anything intrinsic to any of them.

~Sensei

We will now attempt to contemplate the mind. The mind plays a profound role in decision making. Its impact on our food consumption choices is substantial. The only other phenomena that may rival its influence are your emotions. However, the mind has an element of mystery that has led to entire fields of study being created to understand it. What actually is the mind? What truly is its function and power? These questions and more are the focus of this contemplation.

It is important to first make a clear distinction between the mind and the brain. Unfortunately, many people use *mind* and *brain* interchangeably in regular conversation. This is a mistake. It often results in poor decision making and confusion about cause and effect. If you are to transcend the limits of the body, this necessarily includes the brain. Let's take up what we can know about the brain from observation.

The first observation of the brain has to do with location. You can ask the question: Where is the brain? To which you only need to point to your head. Though you may not have ever seen your own brain, it is reasonable to assume that the photos of other peoples' brains, and their location, is similar to your own. This is not a matter of faith but deductive reasoning.

Next, we can inquire about the dimensions of the brain. We can ask how long is the brain? How wide is the brain? This can be easily, and accurately, known by measuring it. Thanks to modern technological advances these measurements can be known about any brain. Likewise, due to the history of actual human brains being measured even prior to modern technological advances, there is plenty of data available regarding the average measurements of the brain. There are plenty of details about this down to age ranges and gender.

We can also ask, and answer: What color is the brain? Likewise, we can inquire about the weight of the brain. The brain is a physical phenomenon. Again, due to human investigation into the brain this has been known for a long time. The point is that any question that can be asked about any physical object can be asked, and answered, about the brain. Probably the most intriguing question about the brain has to do with how it functions. Much is known about its function though there is a lot more to learn.

Let's now inquire about the mind. We will use the same language and questions that we used for the brain. Remember, we are attempting to understand the differences (if any) between brain and mind. The first question for you is: Where is the mind? What is your immediate response to this question? If you are one attached to the self you may respond that the mind is "in the brain." Alternatively, you may just point to your head. Are you sure about this? Consider the question again. **Where** is the mind?

If you state a location for the mind, it presents a big challenge. It means that you know its precise coordinates. We saw with the brain how easy it is to demonstrate its location. Are you able to point to the location of the mind? If you are pointing to the body, does this really answer the question? If you believe the mind is in the head, or anywhere in the body, then you should be able to state its precise location. How is that you are experiencing something (i.e. mind) yet can't state definitively where it is?

The inability to state where the mind is often leads to the use of mind and brain interchangeably in conversation. For example, if you were to begin a sentence with "in my mind I believe…" would this be equivalent to "in my brain I believe" such and such a thing? The second sentence sounds cluttered and somehow does not capture what you are trying to express. Where is the mind? Hopefully, you are beginning to feel the force of this question.

Perhaps trying to locate mind is too difficult. Let's move on to the next question. What are the dimensions of mind? How long is mind? How tall is mind? How wide is mind? These are easy questions to answer regarding the brain. Do you find these measurement questions about mind easier to answer than the location questions about the brain? Or, do you find them equally difficult to answer? Perhaps you may find them even more difficult to answer. It would seem that if the mind is a *thing* or phenomenon that we should be able to easily answer these questions. What is making these questions about measurements so challenging to answer?

Try to answer the color question we asked about the brain. What color is mind? Does this sound like a ridiculous question? Intuitively, it probably does and should. Presently, it may seem you are no closer to understating mind than you were before asking these questions. This will certainly be true if you are attached to the self. But, if you consciously sit with these questions about mind, major openings will arise in your awareness. Here are some things you will directly come to realize.

The apparent paradox is that you are having the experience of mind yet cannot definitely state anything about its physical attributes. How can this be? First, it should be clear that the brain and mind are not synonymous. If you remain unconvinced of this fact you should continue to try to answer the questions raised above until you realize the futility of doing so. As the brain and mind are not synonymous you should refrain from use of language that confuses you, (and others) by using the words interchangeably.

It is easy to understand the intrigue about mind. The paradox seems unresolvable. One way you could approach this is to discard the word mind. That is, discontinue any use of the word *mind* or any reference to it. This too becomes problematic. Although you may remove the word from your vocabulary the experience of mind would still be fully present. The power of mind seems to have little to do with the word itself but rather a particular self-verifiable experience.

Mind has no identifiable location. Wherever you state that mind is would mean that it has coordinates. It has a place. As this is not the case we can definitely say that mind is non-local. Additionally, it is not "over there" or far away. This could be quite difficult to fully grasp if you are attached to self. As it stands, you are simultaneously experiencing a finite measurable phenomenon called brain along with non-measurable non-local mind.

This co-presence presents an even greater paradox for the one attached to selfhood. The manufactured self tends to want to identify with the brain and body. It feels secure. The sense data and habits of the brain are easy to observe and repeat. Whatever habitual patterns mind may reflect they are usually directly related to the body, selfhood and their preservation. But, a being unattached to self-identity is free to choose among the best possibilities. This being knows that mind is not limited to the needs of the body. It can't be starved and it will never become sleepy or thirsty.

Mind can act completely independently of the body. You experience the truth of this on a daily basis. Mind is usually engaged in one of three modes. One, thinking about the past. Second, thinking about the future. Third, and most rare, focused on the present moment. The present moment experience of mind for most is usually not conscious. Meaning present moment of mind usually consciously occurs when there is a perceived threat to selfhood or body. Though this may be a present moment of mind it is unstable due to its catalyst which is fear.

The body and brain must at all times be in one location at a time. It is only mind that is free from the limitation of locality. The body may be sitting in a car or bus but mind can be wrapped up in thoughts about an experience in an entirely different city, state or country. The speed at which mind moves is not matched by any phenomenon except maybe the speed of light. I believe mind is faster than light.

If you are unable to consciously be in the present moment without it being triggered by a perceived harm, you will often make poor decisions about really important matters. Likewise, any sense of peace or continuity of ease will elude you. This is why it's so important to understand the uniqueness of mind when compared to the brain, body and selfhood. It draws your attention to the fact that mind has none of the limitations that the latter three phenomena possess.

There is another phenomenon that you may inadvertently co-mingle with mind. It is easy to confuse *memory* and mind. But, as with body, brain and selfhood, memory also is distinct from mind. You have probably used or heard the phrase " I'm losing my mind." Or maybe you've said that other people have lost their minds. Of course these statements are used in many contexts. One of those contexts is when you can't remember something that you think you ought to easily remember.

I use to do spiritual counseling with patients in a doctor's office. Some patients expressed deep concern about losing their memory. This was mostly expressed by some of the more elderly patients. It was a serious sign of decline to them and caused them a lot of suffering. To forget a grandchild's name, or directions to a place that you still often go to can be frustrating.

When you forget things you've easily remembered for years without effort you feel that you are declining. As many of them would say "I'm losing my mind." This is an uncomfortable feeling. This is not exclusively the experience of senior citizens. Many adults in their 40's begin to experience this. The causes of memory loss are many. I'll now share with you what I use to share with any patient, young or old, when they suffer due to short memory or memory loss.

The mind and memory are not dependent on each other. Memory is an activity of the brain. In fact, modern medicine and science states it knows where memories are stored in the brain. Neuroscientist say they have identified several locations for storing memories depending on the type of memory. That said, they are extremely difficult to track. Given this bit of insight we can clearly establish that mind and memory are not synonymous. At a minimum, memory's location can be determined but mind's cannot.

I now ask you the question I use to ask patients. How is it that you can see (or know) that your memory is fading? What is able to communicate this fact yet itself is not fading along with it? The answer is mind. The notion of losing one's mind is a fiction. The truth is mind can neither be lost or found. You should have already directly observed the truth of the latter part of this statement in this present contemplation. You may now add another observable truth. Mind cannot be lost. Reflect upon this deeply, then continue reading.

It is clear that mind is not constrained in ways that we've observed about the body or brain. However, with that freedom comes one requirement that relates to the body. Mind is free to produce ideas about whatever it wants. But, it needs the body to implement many of those ideas. The irony is that mind is superior to body in every aspect but it cannot act unilaterally in the world. Without the body to implement mind's ideas in the world the ideas essentially remain only possibilities.

The relationship between mind and body is often full of conflicts. The power of the body is deeply connected with self-identity and sense data. The more one is attached to self-identity, body and sense data the more difficult it is for mind to be known purely as it is. Mind has access to the body but it also has access to Consciousness. Mind has the ability to see higher expressions of truth. The body, along with the brain, is limited to those matters that preserve them. This body-brain duo does not exercise discernment but is reactionary.

For example, the body won't give any thought about whether something is healthy if it's hungry. If you put something in your mouth the body will do its best to digest it. It may not always successfully do so but it will try. The desire for the biological organism to live is tied to life itself. The process of life forming over incalculable time has made the unfolding of the bio-process a formidable force. In part, this is why the struggle between mind and body is so intense. You are mutually experiencing the will of life to live along with mind. This is intense co-presence. The body has myriad needs while mind has none.

More often than not, you likely find the self you've manufactured, and the body you experience, prevailing over mind. "Your" mind tells you that such-and-such a thing would be a more prudent or wise way to proceed but is overruled by the self and body. This is particularly true in cases of addiction. More commonly though, this is experienced by the masses of people due to lack of understanding mind. Hence, why we are deeply contemplating mind so intensely. But, why does the influence of self-identity and body seem so much more powerful than mind?

The differences between the power of mind, selfhood and body has nothing to do with anything intrinsic to any of them. It has everything to do with one's awareness and where that awareness is focused. If you are preoccupied with selfhood and body then your awareness will remain stuck in these two phenomena. Occasionally, you may have experiences of not being trapped in these two but without a deeper awakening about the nature of them you'll remain under their dominance. A healthy dose of wisdom must be introduced, and practiced, before there can be any meaningful lasting shifts in you.

When the awareness is directed at a single phenomenon your ability to see into that phenomenon with exceptional clarity dramatically increases. We've been contemplating mind. If you've been paying close attention you probably have noticed how elusive it appears to be. You are able to acknowledge and experience mind, but that seems to be all. You may not be sure if mind *acts alone* or are you driving its activity.

You can discover the answer to this with deeper contemplation. The food of the mind is sense data. This data is presented through the senses. Most people are familiar with what are traditionally called the five senses. The five senses usually refer to sight, touch, smell, taste and hearing. However, there is a sixth sense. The sixth sense is thought.

You can think of sense organs as the mouth. They are the points of entry for all sense data. Sense data is the food. Mind is like the stomach. The activity of mind (i.e. thinking) is a digestive process. Thoughts themselves are the product of all of the above.

On the biological level, no activity of the human body consumes more energy than the process of digesting food. On the level of mind, thinking requires the most energy. Likewise, unlike the body, mind is often in a perpetual state of consumption. That is to say, that sense data is constantly being presented and mind is constantly trying to digest it all. One can decide whether to eat food or not. But, one cannot not decide not to hear a bell ring once the ears have heard it. Nor can the eyes refuse to see a form once seen.

Given the bombardment of sense data, often presented in milliseconds, it may seem nearly impossible to focus awareness on a single phenomenon. Presently, you are contemplating mind and the very nature of thought itself. This you are doing while simultaneously digesting whatever other sense data may be presenting to you. So, it must be the case, that even though this bombardment of sense data may be overwhelming, it is also true that it can be simultaneously observed from a "place" that is not experiencing the overwhelm that is witnessed. You are doing it now.

For any sense data to become proper food for digestion by mind it requires three components. These three are a functioning sense organ, the proper phenomenal object and a meeting between the first two. Consider the following example. The organ in this example is the ear. What does the ear consume? It consumes sound. The ear cannot consume form nor taste nor any other phenomena. Sound is the exclusive phenomenal object for the ear. Not until the ear meets with a sound will there be any sense data fed to mind. The ear and sound are codependent and co-necessary to producing food that will then be digested into a thought (or multiple thoughts) by mind.

Assuming a properly functioning sense organ is accompanied by its corresponding sense object, the formulation of thought may be gradual or immediate. In the case of a loud noise, the immediate thought may be "that is loud." In the case of a symphony playing a set of songs it may be gradual. From the first few notes, you may not like what you hear but by the middle or end of the set you may give a standing ovation. What you should now be able to add to your understanding of mind is that due to sense data, and how quickly it can be presented, you do not have one hundred percent control over mind.

Now is a good time to recap some salient points you have learned about mind through this contemplation. One, mind and brain are not synonymous. Two, mind has no observable physical characteristics and can't be measured. Three, mind has no location or coordinates. Four, while mind cannot be measured, the experience of mind is still clearly evident. Five, removal of the word *mind* from your vocabulary does not eliminate the experience of mind. Six, memory and mind are two different phenomena and should not be conflated. Seven, the activity of mind is inextricably connected to the sense organs and sense data. Eight, one hundred percent control over the mind is not possible, or necessary, in order to master it.

These eight points should be demonstrably self proven from engaging in this contemplation on mind. If not, continue to reflect on any of them until you reach an experiential truth about them. As you engage in deeper contemplations about mind, you may discover the manufactured self wants to find a way to cling to it. Your self wants to take ownership of mind as it attempts to do with the body, nature and the universe. The act of thinking is such an intimate experience that the self wants to digest mind into itself as part of its identity. However, mind nor its content, can ever be *eaten* by the self. This is true even though thoughts may arise in infinite number within mind. Unfortunately, most people struggle to master mind because they are too preoccupied with trying to construct mind's food (thought) into a self.

As you don't have complete dominion over the experience of mind, how can it be tamed or mastered? Mind seems impossible to corner. Conversely, mind can corner the self any time it wishes to do so. Have you noticed this in your experience? Mind can cause you to run the same loop of thoughts, or a singular thought, for hours days or years. What is often called *trauma* is really a thought that one feels unable to escape. It is a thought about a particular moment, or series of events, that is deposited into the memory to which selfhood clings.

There is a way to master mind without having complete control over its many facets. Mind mastery, for the purposes of this contemplation, refers to the ability not to suffer your thoughts. There is a conscious way of not clinging to the product (i.e. thoughts) of mind. The way to achieve this may surprise you. It is not by attempting to tackle mind and subdue it. How can the experience of mind, with all of its peculiar "characteristics" we have acknowledged, ever be conquered? It cannot.

It was previously stated that mind can produce so many thoughts that the self can never get to the end of them. Focusing on subduing mind is like focusing on eliminating the smoke rather than the actual issue which is the fire. Mind cannot be discovered. It cannot be owned. It cannot be managed. Furthermore, unlike nature and the universe, mind shares no constituent physical components with body. Nor does it share any **physical** component with nature or the universe. There is only one *thing* that mind shares in common with body, nature and the universe. That will be addressed in the 6th contemplation on Consciousness.

Another key observation about mind is important to note here. Not only do the sense organs constantly present a nonstop stream of sense data, but this mind-food most often is recycled. What does this mean? *Recycling* refers to the cyclical reoccurrence of sense data that has already been served to the mind but never fully digested. **This** is how mind is able to corner the self. This is part of how the sense of overwhelm arises.

Undigested thoughts are perhaps even more harmful than undigested food. When you don't fully digest your food there will inevitably be a problem experienced in the body. These problems will be mild to severe depending on how long this continues. Undigested food is normally stored as fat or other harmful material in the body. Likewise, undigested thoughts recycle through mind repeatedly. This recycling matter deserves further observation,

How many thoughts today have you recycled? That is, how many times has the same thought, or some version of it, reoccurred today? Something someone said. A lyric you heard on the radio today or years ago. What you want to eat today. What you did eat today. Something you saw online. Closely observing this recycling phenomenon for a single day will experientially demonstrate the truth about the existence of un-recycled thoughts.

One might ask this logical question. How can one stop the recycling of ideas? How can an idea be fully digested? This is a deep mind and self-mastery question. Again, trying to stop or capture ideas themselves is a futile endeavor. The best way to be unaffected by undigested ideas is not to grasp or cling on to them. If a repetitive thought keeps

coming back don't say " I must stop thinking this thought."
Likewise, don't ask why it is you keep having this thought.
Let it arise, abide and decline. It will be your lack of attention and awareness on it that will naturally make it subside
or stop all together. Try it.

This non-clinging and non-grasping technique can
prove extremely valuable when it comes to food cravings
and eating habits. Food cravings are a natural reoccurring
phenomenon. The human biology seemingly has a technology of its own. When it needs or wants foods it has many different ways of notifying you. Impulsive eating and overeat-
ing often result from these signals. Many people can not re-
sist even the slightest onset of a feeling of hunger. As soon
as hunger on any level is detected they want to eat something and most often do it.

Food cravings are a natural part of the human biological experience. However, there are at least two things you
should know about food cravings. First, they can be overrid-
den. Second, natural biological food cravings are not the
same as the artificial food cravings you most often experience and act upon. A still mind is able to see these truths
quite clearly. As you may self-identify with the body, and
your awareness is habitually preoccupied with the body, the
wisdom of mind remains somewhat veiled from you.

It's important to distinguish between natural food
cravings and artificial food cravings. This distinction can be
clearly observed by mind. This is because unlike the manufactured self the mind is not attached to either type. Co-presence is deeply at work here. Artificial food cravings shall be
addressed first.

Artificial food cravings, like self-identity, is manufactured. It is a false call for energy by the body. These artificial cravings are driven by *the four horsemen*. The four
horsemen of artificial food cravings are taste buds, tradition,

culture and habit. A deep sense of selfhood is essential for these horsemen to be effective. These each play a role on one's thoughts about food choices and the corresponding eating habits produced.

Taste buds are non other than conductors of a particular type of sense data. That is to say *flavor*. If your tongue palette is not polluted, it is capable of recognizing 5 different types of flavor. The five flavors include salty, sour, bitter, sweet and umami. Many people have a preference for salty and sweet tastes. This is particularly true of anyone who consumes a conventional western diet. These diets are usually high in salt, sugar and fat.

The five flavors are detected by specific regions of the tongue. Salty tastes are detected at the tip of the tongue. Sweet tastes are experienced at the point halfway between the tip of the tongue and middle of the tongue. Umami tastes, sometimes called savory, are detected in the middle of the tongue. Bitter tastes are detected at the back of the tongue. Sour tastes are detected on the right and lefts sides of the tongue.

A great deal of weight is given to how food tastes when deciding what to eat. This is natural. No one wants to eat food that does not taste good. However, taste buds are easily manipulated. If the palette is bombarded with salty, sweet or oily foods it will desire those types of foods. Other foods not high in salt or sugar content will seem bland or tasteless. Take note of the foods you seem to "prefer." Are you able to identify the dominant flavor of those foods?

The good news is that due to taste buds being easily trainable you can break the chains of attachment they create. For example, if you are addicted to sugar or believe you have a *sweet tooth* you should know that this is a myth. Not that you don't experience the craving for sweet things, but that it's actually **you** craving the sugar is untrue. There is a particular fungus in the gut called candida. It's a type of yeast. When candida is out of balance (i.e. overfed) it sends signals to the brain to satiate its cravings. Guess what candida thrives on? It thrives on sugar.

Choosing foods based primarily, or exclusively, on taste buds can prove to be catastrophic for your health. Of the four horsemen, taste buds are probably the most difficult to discover. The taste buds are deeply wrapped up into self-identity. This is what causes you to add extra salt to your food, or sugar to your drink, before even tasting it. You believe you're making these decisions but in reality you're not.

Tradition is another horseman that participates in the generation of artificial food cravings. This is one of two horsemen that asserts itself on the social level of existence. The self-identified being desires permanence. Permanence among phenomena is not possible. Tradition, in relation to food consumption, gives the self a bit of false security. The health value of the food is irrelevant. There is pride in feeling that you are carrying on a tradition of eating this particular food (or dish) that may go back several generations or thousands of years. To cease continuing this tradition is unthinkable. What foods do you presently eat based in large part, or primarily, upon some tradition?

There is deep fear in the one attached to the manufactured self about not participating in traditions. This is true even where those traditions are unhealthy. Herd mentality is simply a consensus among self attached beings. The prospect of being the one to rise above tradition, or establish a healthier version of it, feels too risky for most people. Non-participation in the tradition may be deemed a rejection of the herd. This could lead to being ostracized by the herd.

Culture, like tradition, is also expressed on the social level. This horseman carries even more persuasive power about food choices and practices than tradition does. It is one thing to abstain from participation in a tradition. But, where food and culture are intertwined with self-identity, any departure from the cultural norm is seen as a slight against the entire group and its history. People will go so far as to call into question your entire identity if you don't eat certain foods because you're operating on a deeper level of consciousness.

It's inevitable that as you shed attachment to self-identity, and make more conscious food choices, that some foods associated with the culture to which others identify you with will be eliminated. On numerous occasions, I have had the experience of others looking at me in amazement and even suspicion. They would ask me "so you never eat such and such food…not even on such and such holiday?" It's almost as though they felt they could not connect with me because the cultural food component was not shared. Having deeper consciousness about eating choices often makes culturally entangled individuals feel uncomfortable.

Their discomfort usually expresses itself in aversion to you, a friendly uneasiness or strong affirmation in continuing to eat the way they presently do. For example, "well I don't know about you but I'm going to have some burgers, hot dogs and a milkshake today at the bbq." Or they may say something like "great don't eat it…that means more for me!" Another common cultural retort is "it was good enough for your grandparents and myself but it's not good enough for you now?" Then there are the classics "I believe in a balanced approach to nutrition" and " I believe everything in moderation is fine." What foods are you continuing to eat due to cultural persuasion and mere acquiescence?

Habit is also a highly influential horseman. Habit plays out on the level of body. Specifically, it involves the brain. Due to its finite characteristics the brain is highly susceptible to initiating habitual behavior. Once stuck on any given loop it will continue to run that loop until it is specifically overwritten. It cannot self overwrite. That power belongs to mind. Once a habitual pattern, like choosing unhealthy foods, has been repeated enough it becomes nearly unconscious behavior. Again, we look at the habit of adding salt or sugar to something before tasting it. This habit rides along with taste buds and before you know it a deadly addiction is being created.

Not all habits are bad but at some point still do become unconscious acts. Once a false craving by the body is created you immediately seek to satisfy it. This despite an awareness that this particular habit is counter to good health. On the other hand, all good habits are conscious. This is because the ever-aware remain cognizant at all times as to why they've chosen one option over another. These good habits then transform into a lifestyle approach. Once good habits reach the level of lifestyle they can have the feeling of being unconscious. But, they actually remain conscious simply because the mind has taken over decision making rather than the manufactured self, sense data, body or brain. We can now take up natural food cravings.

A natural food craving is the biological organism (here the body) expressing a real need for energy. It is expressing the need for energy to carry out essential processes needed to continue the life of the organism. It is important that natural food cravings not be exclusively limited to eating food as you presently understand food to be. Bio-beings must have ample and appropriate energy specifically helpful to their particular lifeforms. The four horsemen play no role in natural food cravings. This is because natural food cravings precede them. Natural food cravings arise out of interdependence of phenomena created by the phenomenon called *life*.

Earlier in this contemplation on mind, the digestive process was mentioned. One of the fascinating facts about digestion is that part of the energy of the food being consumed is used to digest that same food. Anywhere from 15-25% of the energy of the food being consumed is used to digest that food. Digestion definitely qualifies as a natural food craving of the body.

Another natural food (i.e energy) craving is sunlight. The sun provides vitamin D and impacts serotonin levels in the body. Perhaps, you live in a region where there is very little sun. Alternatively, maybe you've experienced no sunlight for an extended period of time. What happened to your energy level when the sun emerged? It likely increased. The abundance of sunlight is one of the major driving factors of the global tourism industry. People are literally willing to pay to be fed by the sun. They know how good it makes them feel.

Next, we can acknowledge sleep as a natural food craving of the human body. Lack of proper sleep can ultimately lead to chronic diseases. These include weakening of the immune system, high blood pressure and diabetes. Sleep deprivation can also result in problems as serious as heart attacks and strokes. Lack of sleep has also been shown to reduce sex drive.

You will note that lack of sleep-food wreaks havoc on the brain. It impairs the ability to think. It causes brain fog and memory loss as well as makes learning anything exponentially more difficult. Likewise, the body suffers dearly from lack of sleep-food. Fatigue, lethargy, emotional imbalances as well as crankiness all become more prevalent due to lack of sleep-food.

One of the clearly observable facts about human biology is movement. Movement seems to be an essential component to this bio-being's expression of life. In fact, it is well known that insufficient movement of the body often results in atrophy of muscles or important systems. Likewise, the energy levels decrease significantly when the body is too sedentary for extended periods. Diseases such as obesity and circulation problems can arise as a result of not moving the body enough.

Movement of any sort requires energy. You may note that your muscles become more tight if you do not stretch or move enough. Even in young people, lack of movement can be extremely damaging. While their muscles may maintain some degree of flexibility their lack of movement will ultimately result in the previously mentioned problems. For example, their cardiovascular strength will become quite poor. There are many young adults, and teens, whom due to their sedentary lifestyles struggle to run a single lap around a track, swim a few laps in a pool or walk a couple of miles without extreme difficulty. Many can't do any of these things at all.

We see that movement-food also qualifies as a natural food craving. Like all of the previously mentioned natural food cravings (including sleep) movement not only increases energy but also uses energy. Depending on the activity, as little as a few calories to several hundred calories may be burned. The need to move is self-verifiable. If you've ever had to sit or stand for an extended period of time it can become extremely uncomfortable. You may have also observed how mothers all over the world rock their children in a rhythmic motion to comfort their child who may be distressed or crying. The importance of movement-food cannot be overstated.

If we are going to discuss natural food cravings, we must obviously mention conventional food. Food **can** be a source of energy. But, as has been noted previously in the discussion about artificial food cravings, many foods deplete the body of energy. Commensurate with the evolution of nature and life, food from the earth has been an essential source of energy. Many grains, vegetables and fruits have been made available in such a way that one could literally "live off of the land." The type, quality and quantity of the food consumed determines its real energy value.

It is interesting to note that while the brain and body suffer dearly from the lack of any of the natural foods, mind only suffers from the lack of one of them. That is spiritual-food. Spiritual-food are those thoughts that bring harmony and balance into your experience. Mind is in constant need of producing spiritual-food until the attachment to self-identity is broken. Similar to eating unhealthy foods that negatively impact the physical body, ignorance about spiritual-food will not be a defense to the results (i.e. mental pain and suffering) for being deficient in it.

It takes a discerning eye to see the level of subtlety at play in regards to spiritual-food. You must not mistake the biological responses of sickness, diseases or physical pain as the only signs of spiritual-food malnutrition. No, there are far more subtle antecedent phenomena that are proper signs of spiritual-food malnutrition. Some examples include: poor decision making, disharmonious relationships, overwhelming doubt, frequent anxiety and remaining stuck in the past or fearful of the future.

There are many more types of spiritual-food malnutrition. There's no need to list them all. From the above listed examples you should be able to understand the nature and flavor of them. Physical symptoms are more obvious to you only because of your attachment to body-identity. Each type of natural food previously mentioned has its own unique energy source. Spiritual-food is no exception. For spiritual-food that source is Consciousness itself.

If indeed Consciousness itself is the source for spiritual-food, how do you consume it? To energize the biology, one can consume various liquids, fruits, vegetables and grains to get sufficient vitamins and minerals. For sleep-food, rest is the source and so on. But, how does one consume something like Consciousness that lacks any tangible "garden?" Where does Consciousness grow? Does it also have an energy source? How could you really know the answers to these questions?

These types of questions, and all similar to these, are yet another example of spiritual-food deprivation. A mind run amok and filled with questions that either seem (1) unanswerable or (2) without end are signs that spiritual-food is lacking. With sufficient spiritual-food you become stable and calm. You recognize that all questions have an *answer* but also that knowing those answers may be unnecessary. There are many healthy foods one can eat to live a long healthy life. It is not necessary, nor perhaps even possible, for you to consistently eat them all even in a single lifetime. Spiritual-food is the same. In fact, if you could fully digest only a handful of spiritual-food your mind could be satiated for life.

Consider the following questions which are indicative of spiritual-food malnutrition. Do I have enough? Will I have enough? Am I enough? You've perhaps asked these questions. If not, perhaps you have wondered what will your future be like? How long will you live? How will you die? You will note that sleep-food, movement-food and the rest are not sufficient in and of themselves to answer these types of questions. These questions can only be fully satiated by spiritual-food.

Earlier the question was raised as to how to consume Consciousness. We will be taking up Consciousness in the next contemplation. I trust that after that contemplation you'll be in a clearer state to come back to this question. I also trust that if you have followed and understood enough of what has been explored in this present contemplation on mind, in conjunction with the previous four contemplations, that you'll arrive at a harmonious answer about spiritual-food and its source which is Consciousness. We now proceed to the contemplation on Consciousness.

CONTEMPLATION 6: Consciousness

In my early days of spiritual seeking I set a high standard. I said that the destination, not the journey, is what matters most.

~Sensei

Consciousness is intriguing. Exploring it can be both perplexing and literally enlightening. That said, our contemplation on Consciousness will remain focused and closely associated with the subject matter of this book. We have been exploring what an enlightened being (i.e. you in your highest awareness) would take into consideration about eating. It's important to understand this point. We are exploring the thought process and influences of spiritual reasoning about food choices, not about what you ought to eat. You are getting an insider view into one being's (mine) contemplations without obstruction. So, rather than explore Consciousness as an "it" or "thing" we will simply seek to detect the presence of Consciousness in this contemplation.

I ask you to reflect upon this fundamental question. Why is there something rather nothing? That is, why is there anything at all rather than nothing at all? You must focus here and not let your mind get distracted by subsequent or tangential thoughts. Why is there something rather than nothing? This question is not concerned with "how things are" or "what things are." In fact, it's not even a question about things. A question about any of these aspects comes after addressing the one we've just taken up.

I spent years looking for an answer to this question. I read more books than I can recall and had numerous conversations with intelligent and spiritual people as part of my process. My investigation into this certainly bore fruit. I explored this question from myriad scientific, religious, mythological, philosophical and spiritual perspectives. I was only interested in Truth without allegiance to or discrimination against the source.

If you'd like to explore this question on your own it may prove to be a worthwhile endeavor. That said, the purpose of one sharing wisdom with others is hopefully to provide a more direct route to full-realization and knowing. So allow me to share with you. I learned about many wonderful ideas and origin stories. Many of these insights have served as jewels for me along the way. Throughout my life, which has been nearly singularly focused on spiritual clarity and self-mastery, I was able to understand how and why many of these ideas arose in Consciousness.

The single most important wisdom that I arrived at forced me back to the question. I finally realized that this question **cannot** be answered with a who, what, when, where or how response. As fascinating as these answers can be, they all miss the mark when trying to answer this particular *why* question. Why is there something rather than nothing? Let's take a closer look at the reasons why **all** verbal responses are insufficient to answer our question.

This question is often answered by explaining "who" created things, the world or all things that exists. Many cultures have origin stories about how their people or country came to be. These explanations often involve a plethora of deities and or a single supreme deity. In short, things were created by particular gods or one God. Despite the seemingly unending chaos and strife of the present day, it is still statistically true that the vast majority of human beings believe in some form of deity or deities. So for these people a who-response is their answer to the question.

Somehow, the belief that there is a supreme deity, or a number of them, responsible for this creation relieves the minds of those who believe this. One can find some solace through faith. The existential value of faith cannot be over-stated. Often life simply makes no sense. Try as you will to understand a particular phenomenon like indiscriminate violence and it feels nearly impossible to do. However, the belief that a supreme power or divinity is always at work allows many to bare life's challenges a bit more easily.

While this *who*-response may provide "an answer" it still seems not to be quite on the mark. Interestingly, if one were to ask: Why is this tea cup on the counter rather than in the cabinet? A perfectly logical answer could be because so-and-so took it out of the cabinet and left it there. For the less discerning mind, it would appear that this question, and its answer, is completely analogous to the our original question: Why is there something rather than nothing? Answer: because so-and-so deity. I trust if you contemplate this deeply you will discover for yourself whether a *who*-response sufficiently answers either question.

Many have answered our question with a *what*-response. A what response is no less problematic than a *who*-response to our question. A *what*-response often can also compound one's confusion when seeking to answer our question. How so? Those not well practiced in contemplative work, on the level and scale at which we are presently engaged, often conflate *what* and *who* into one. They will literally begin to answer the question with a *who*-response. As they explain their response, they then begin to engage in *who-what* responses using both terms interchangeably.

An example of this type of response may sound a bit like the following. "Well the scriptures/oracles/traditions say that so-and-so deity/deities willed such-and-such (or felt such-and-such about a particular people or matter) and as result of that the world (or this land/country/humans) after X period of time came to be. Juxtapose this answer to our question: Why is there something rather than nothing? Are you able to observe the conflation of who and what?

Furthermore, are you able to see how a *what*-response to our question, even without conflating it with *who*, is not sufficient as an answer? If not, this analogy of a *what*-response can help you. Question: Why is this ink red? Answer: Because of color. The answer responds with a what. (i.e. color) Does this answer the question asked? Is anything a particular color because something called color exists? The mind may attempt to assimilate this into a coherent and acceptable answer. But this attempt to massage the *what*-response into an acceptable answer is indicative of a lack of organic internal coherence. For the purposes of our question a *what*-response still misses the mark.

Could a *when*-response answer our question? A *when*-response is exclusively relevant only to time. Any answer to our question that begins with when has strayed far from what is being asked. As it relates to our question, a *when*-response is completely irrelevant. It's more likely to result in tangents that take you further away from a cogent answer. In an attempt to answer this question, you must dispense with beginning with any notion of when. A *when*-response will only obstruct you from what's really being asked and thwart attempts to see something more subtle. The same is true for any *where*-response that could be offered.

We proceed now to a *how*-response to our question. Often *how*-responses get conflated with a *what*-response. A popular example of a *how*-response is a scientific theory. The Big Bang theory is believed by many to explain how the universe began or was created. Some who subscribe to this belief think that this *how*-response (i.e Big Bang Theory) sufficiently answers our question of why there is something rather than nothing. Though this theory, and others similar to it, may not seem as supernatural as other origin stories it nonetheless is an origin story. The difference primarily being Big Bang is "backed or proven" by science rather than by faith.

Nonetheless, to answer our question with a *how-what* response also falls short of sufficiently answering the question. Question:Why is there something rather than nothing? Answer: An immense massive solid mass warmed up to an incredible temperature and then exploded into uncountable pieces in multiple directions etc etc… Imagine if someone were to knock on your door and you asked "why are you here?" If that person answered "I caught a taxi to get here" would that be answering the why? Clearly it would not. The most generous allowance of any *how, what, when, where* response to this *why* question will always be insufficient because they all begin at some point **after** which we are presently inquiring.

What I have ultimately realized is that the question presented in this contemplation is a direct one about Consciousness itself. Why is there something rather than nothing? The answer to this question can only be arrived at experientially. As wonderful, convincing or plausible as any response to this question may be, they all necessarily miss the mark because of their starting points. When do all articulations of any response begin? My contemplation on this revealed to me that at some point (no matter how near or remote) **after** Consciousness. This means that a *why*-response would also fall short of adequately answering our question.

What do I mean by all articulations begin after Consciousness? Allow this analogy involving music and musical notes. If you listen to a piano being played, so long as your ears are functioning well enough you will hear the notes. (i.e. sounds) For the vast majority of human beings, hearing the sounds is all they'll be able to do. Perhaps they may also have an opinion about what they're hearing. They can state whether they like or dislike it but not much more than this.

A significantly smaller group of beings listening to this same piano being played will be able to detect more than the former group. This group can state what chords and notes are actually being played. For example, they are able to distinguish a C major chord versus another chord like D minor. This is because their ear consciousness vocabulary is more robust, refined and experienced than the former group. This is likely due to some deeper exposure to music and experience with the piano in particular.

There are an infinitesimal number of beings who are aware of the sounds, the notes and chords but also the silence. In fact, these extremely rare beings know, experientially, that the silence (i.e. absence of sound) is essential to being able to hear anything at all. This silence of which I speak may only seem momentary…like a millisecond before the next note. But, the fully aware being knows that without this *perpetual silent note* that no other notes could be heard. There is a universal note that was, is and remains before, during and after the playing of any audible note.

The first group of listeners are like those individuals who eat but don't understand what they are eating or why. They can only state the name of the food (i.e. burger) and whether they like the taste or not. The second group of listeners are like those who could not only name what they are eating but also the ingredients, nutritional value or constituent parts of what they are eating. They may likely have a scientific background or specialized understanding of conventional food but not of the phenomenon called food. That is, they are only able to describe what is perceptible to their senses.

The third group of listeners are those rare beings who understand the entire phenomenon of food and the purpose of eating. These beings may also have some technical knowledge of food or none at all. For the being that understands a phenomenon on its most fundamental level, the myriad expressions or varieties of it, are of minor interest if at all. Experientially, these beings know that the various expressions of a phenomenon do not increase or decrease the phenomenon itself.

Please reflect deeply on this music and piano analogy as it relates to understanding Consciousness. The last observation about this analogy I'd like to share with you will shuttle you further along in this contemplation. Think of hearing a note as a moment of "mind consciousness" and the perpetual silence before, during and after each note as Consciousness itself. When you hear a note, and attach an opinion to it (e.g. like or dislike) this is just like the false-self to which you habitually listen to and cling. This phantom-self is solely an extended moment of mind consciousness. Like all notes the self will be played and then fade away. You may wonder to where. A slight clue: where do the musical notes go after you can no longer hear them? Stay with this train of thought until the answer reveals itself experientially.

To close out this particular contemplation, I'll mention the best way I believe to know Consciousness. As a general matter, do not seek to understand Consciousness but rather to **know** it. Merely seeking to understand Consciousness will result in circular travel for an incalculable span of time. Undoubtedly, many true seekers of wisdom and truth are stuck in this cycle precisely because they seek to understand rather than to know. Seekers often lure themselves into thinking that they are getting closer to an answer. Although they have not reached a definitive knowing, they find that perpetual searching can be extremely insightful and invigorating. This is especially true if their intentions are pure.

Conventional cliches such as "the journey is more important than the destination" or "the questions are more important than the answers" are statements I fully reject. It seems that such statements are only really acceptable when it comes to spiritual matters. In no other area of life would you find such statements agreeable. Imagine you scheduled a flight from your home country to another country on the opposite side of the globe. It would not be acceptable to you if the pilot landed in a country half way to your destination and then stated, "well I did not take you where you wanted to go but it was a nice flight."

In my early days of spiritual seeking I set a high standard. I said that the destination, not the journey, is what matters most. I must know…and I will know. Fidelity to that standard saved me a lot of grief. Perhaps I did miss out on some additional experiences but I had plenty of meaningful and impactful experiences staying true to this standard. I wanted an experiential answer to every question I had. My standard allowed me to be free from concern from the thoughts, beliefs or critiques of all of those who did not understand or agree with my life decisions.

I never loss sight of my standard or the destination. Thankfully, I did arrive. I have no more questions as they have all been experientially answered in various ways. They were not always enjoyable and at times were outright excruciating. Every moment along the way was necessary given the magnitude of what I was inquiring about, and how determined I was to know and not merely understand. I remained faithful and was rewarded with the experiential answers that my particular karmic makeup required.

People often think it is a display of hubris or arrogance to state having "arrived" when speaking of spiritual matters. In my case, my arrival has to do with reaching a particular shore. I do not claim to know it all. Nor did I ever seek to know it all. I only sought to understand the quintessential and most relevant aspects of my particular inquiries. Admittedly, this took a significant amount of time. In fact, it took decades of my life. Still, I stayed on the path knowing that if my inquiries were one hundred percent answered that it would be worth whatever experience I had to endure in order to know.

Some beings are willing to see a particular matter through to its conclusion or destination no matter the cost. I count myself among them at least in regards to my spiritual path. Jobs, various types of relationships and myriad other experiences I was willing to part with (or completely miss) if only I could reach my destination. I had no idea so many years ago that my spiritual questions would have any connection or impact whatsoever on my eating practices. But, they did. It is one of the main catalyst for me deciding to write this book. This book, like so many other events in my life, are not ones I intentionally set out to experience. I simply embraced them all as part of the fullness of the unfolding of my karma.

As it regards my inquiry into Consciousness, I'll share with you the three most powerful and effective parameters I believe lead to a true knowing of it. First, you should inquire without allegiance to words or their sources. Second, remove all attachments to a sense of selfhood. Third, don't rely on thoughts alone. These three parameters should be applied to any method of spiritual inquiry you decide to implement. You'll discover that they will squeeze out every ounce of unnecessary activity required to directly know Consciousness. Let's look at each one in more detail.

What does it mean to inquire without allegiance to words or their sources? I've had many conversations in my life with people about spiritual matters. Whether assisting a family member or friend, counseling a client or teaching one of my students, I have observed how words often get in the way of direct experiential knowing. The words themselves are not the blame. Words are like all other phenomena. Meaning, they are dependent upon other phenomena, impermanent and empty. (i.e. lack a substantial existence)

When you become attached to the meaning or origin of words it automatically limits what you can know.

An example of obstruction to knowing caused by attachment to a word's meaning or origin can be illustrated in the following manner. Person A believes in an omnipotent God. This person also believes that this God's words have been recorded in a particular book. One line in this scripture states that God has said "don't steal." One can assume that God had some reason for instructing against stealing. God may also then go on to say the negative outcomes of stealing which may also include punishment by this God. Person A believes in this command because he or she believes that "God said so."

Let's change the source of the statement "don't steal" to that of a thief. A person who is known for regularly stealing things from others is often heard telling other people that stealing is not a good idea. Person A might reject such words from this source due to the inability to see past what they perceive to be a hypocrite. How many people would dismiss the advice of this thief based upon the source? Wouldn't a thief know from direct experience the dangers and risks of stealing from others better than one who has never stolen anything? Would you give "God's word" more truth value than a thief in this scenario? If so, why? Answer: unnecessary attachment to the word's meaning or source of it. Remain open to Truth being revealed from non-preferred, unfamiliar or seemingly contradictory sources.

The second parameter to be implemented when inquiring into Consciousness is to remove any attachment to selfhood. The first chapter in this book is an extensive contemplation on self-identity and its vicissitudes. Some people really struggle with the first parameter of my recommended trio. They have such deep cultural, religious, political or gender based attachments that they can only believe or accept words from particular sources. In my case, I had very little challenges with this. As a voracious reader, the world of ideas is one vast sea to me. Therefore, the attachments I once held were easily broken. That said, it was the attachment to selfhood that was the most challenging standard for me to meet.

I believe that it was my deep attachment to selfhood that unnecessarily prolonged my spiritual inquiries. This also exposed me to dreadfully painful psychological and emotional states that could have been completely avoided. It is no exaggeration to state that my previous attachment to self artificially inflated my process for two decades. Over that period, I was slowly and steadily chipping the self attachment away. But, once I arrived at my intended destination I realized how much effort and energy it took me to keep a sense of self intact.

All of my years of martial arts training, meditation, fasting, prayer, reading, silence and related spiritual exercises were largely aimed at dismantling this attachment to a self. What is often referred to as *life* for me is a meditation. Once the selfhood was shed I arrived at the wisdom of *life as meditation*. There is no point at which I am outside of it. Meditation is life and life is meditation. Every thought, action or word spoken is part of my unbroken karmic expression. The freedom and peace that comes with knowing this is so wonderful that it's beyond articulation.

The third parameter mentioned previously is not to rely on thought alone. People suffer dearly from their thoughts. Personally, I believe this is the primary source of suffering of any sort. It is common in our time to name every type of suffering and seek a separate remedy for each one. However, the power of practicing Chan, meditation, silence and martial arts has shown me quite clearly that all suffering is due to thoughts. I have had moments in martial arts training that I found myself asking "how are you still standing?" Or, "how are you able to endure this?"

When every muscle in my body felt like it was failing or wanted to give up, I had to retreat completely into Consciousness. The more authentically I was able to do so, the more feint the physical sensations of strain or pain became. At other times, they simply were not felt at all. Likewise, in my deepest states of meditation I have had similar experiences. There is an awareness of the body but there is no focus on it. The thoughts stop inquiring or evaluating the body and its sensations. Instead the body just becomes so muted that the awareness has no more interest in it over any other phenomenon. This is true equanimity. This is superior to any form of happiness. It is complete contentment.

Some may wonder if it is actually possible not to rely entirely on thought. There are many powerful techniques for doing this. Martial arts training, silence, fasting and meditation practice are just a few of them. Contemplative practice is also another powerful tool. If you've made it this far into this book, you have a much deeper understanding of what contemplative practice feels like. Fasting, breathing exercises, chanting, prayer and so many other techniques if done correctly (and used for their original intended purposes) can aid one in knowing Consciousness experientially. It's been a pleasure over the years teaching people how to do this and observing their organic realizations.

It is important to note here that thoughts are not bad or good. Bad and good are simply judgements and attachment to two concepts. The reason I made it part of my tri-part guidelines is because it forces a new ability to spring forth. You use your thoughts as a raft and then transcend them. What is there beyond the thoughts in your head? How do you tap into an experiential answer to that question? It begins by realizing the value of thoughts but simultaneously realizing their limitations. The limitations of thought are all observable. The question then becomes: "Observable by what?" (not "who")

*What is the actual relationship between the phenomenon I
call my-self compared with the phenomenon of food?*

~Sensei

Buddha is a Sanskrit word meaning a fully awakened
or enlightened being. This should not be understood as an
"other worldly" being or deity. Rather, the only meaningful
difference between yourself and a buddha is that a buddha
has awakened to the truth of all phenomena. This being is
not trapped in the dream of delusion called self-hood. Therefore, such a being's decisions, way of life and reasoning are
all markedly distinct from other beings.

The title of this book is *Eat Like A Buddha*. Did you
note there were no nutritional guidelines or medical studies
cited? Further, did you notice that there were no recommen-
dations about diets? There was no mention made of carni-
vore versus herbivore, plant-based (or vegan) versus keto or
vegetarian versus pescatarian. Likewise, no guidelines regarding caloric intake, how much protein you need and the
best source of protein are anywhere addressed. This was all
intentional.

The above are all conventional self-centric data points
that will never allow one to arrive at an experiential answer
to the questions this book implicitly raises. Behind the title
of this book are several important questions. What is food?
Why do I make the food choices I do? How would my best
self (i.e. fully aware) spiritually reason about what to eat?
What **ultimate** significance do my eating habits have? What

is the actual relationship between the phenomenon I call my-self compared with the phenomenon of food and eating?

Furthermore, you will also note that I made no appeal to persuade you via Buddhist authorities or sutras. (i.e. scriptural text) Nonetheless, your contemplative results, may align with several Buddhist teachings. If they do, that would be due to your own self-verified truth. For example, the belief that there is no self. This is clearly, though not exclusively, a Buddhist concept. Yet, arrival at this wisdom can be achieved strictly through focused contemplation without invoking Buddhism. The power of **real** contemplative work is that whatever realizations that materialize will be ones that you have personally produced. Later, you may learn other beings have had some of the same realizations. The truth value of those realizations would be self-derived not borrowed.

We've arrived at the final contemplation of this book. You have been presented with several substantial contemplations. I know that if you take each one of them seriously you will discover major life changing truths that will directly impact your eating habits. Given that these contemplations are so intricate I believe there would be great value in making explicit some of the more subtle contemplations within these that are very easy to miss. I'll not present these hidden gems in any particular order. I don't want you to think that any one of them are more important than any other.

If you are unaccustomed to thinking on a fundamental level, the results of your contemplative practice will vary. What is meant by *thinking on a fundamental level*? It has a lot to do with thinking and reflecting minus attachment to a sense of self. That is, the same habitual thoughts you presently engage with would have a completely different impact if you could cease grasping and clinging to a self-perceiver. A valiant attempt has been made to methodically disentangle you from selfhood via these contemplations.

Undoubtedly, one of the previous six contemplations may resonate more with you than another. This is fine. I've written this book knowing that this would likely be the case. To the degree you are able to fully realize, and experientially verify any of the contemplations, the others will open up to you in ways unimaginable. My process in presenting the contemplations was to begin with the self you identify as and slowly move "outward" through the perceived other.

Each contemplation, beginning with the so-called self, all the way to Consciousness itself, was meant to create a direct experience of your real relationship to them. By stopping the habitual thinking about these experiences you are given the opportunity to see Truth as it is. You have the opportunity to observe, on a fundamental level, something that has evaded you up until this point. The cumulative result of practicing these contemplations repeatedly will result in a reversal of your most deeply erroneous views about food and Consciousness. In this state of freedom, you can now approach the question: "How shall I eat?" from a place of knowing and complete wisdom. I trust that deciding from this state of consciousness you will make changes to your eating habits that will free your mind and heal the world. What those changes will be are for you to decide.

I'll now list some of the contemplations that were likely missed. You may find a deep rejection arise to these contemplations. Something in you will say "this does not make sense." Or perhaps "these things have nothing to do with one another." This is simply your sense of personhood trying to keep you from taming and transcending it. Still, don't view this self you have erected as an enemy. Rather accept that as part of Consciousness and body dancing to-gether that a false sense of self could potentially arise. Let it be. Press forward with the contemplation. That self will be forced to quiet itself.

The focus of my style of contemplative work is to reflect deeply on the co-presence of two or more phenomena simultaneously existing. I call this Co-present Contemplation. Your mind has made many assumptions and drawn myriad conclusions due to habitual thinking. You likely habitually conflate several phenomena without discerning their differences or separate phenomena while missing what they actually share. This habitual thinking is fed from data observed through the six senses.

Due to this pattern of habitual thinking, my Co-present Contemplation method builds on this pattern rather than try to break it. However, what is introduced for contemplation pairs are unusual. The unusual co-presence of the phenomena used for this contemplative method forces considerations that you've likely never given much thought to. You'll see from the following contemplations that were embedded in the contemplations of this book. Good luck…

1. What is the relationship between self and:

    a) non-self   f) security   k) Consciousness

    b) other   g) belief

    c) colors   h) sound

    d) weather   i) life

    e) matter   j) multiplicity

2. What is the relationship between food and:

    a) conflict   f) existence   k) Consciousness

    b) time   g) birth

    c) freedom   h) death

    d) sentience   i) movement

    e) intelligence j) opposites

9 798378 056705